Women'sHealth

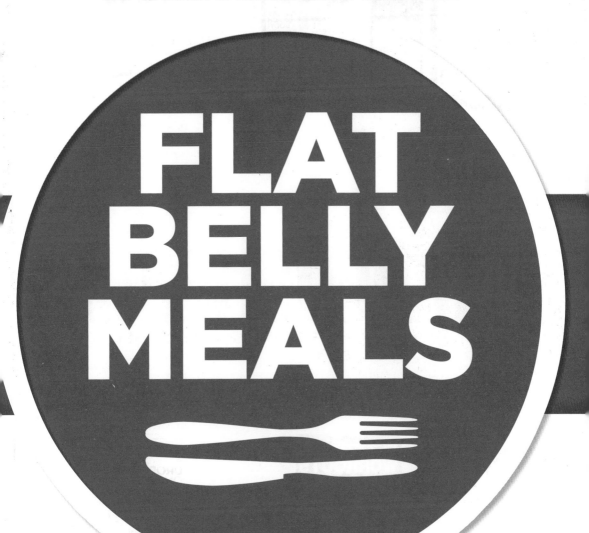

FLAT
BELLY
MEALS

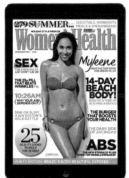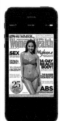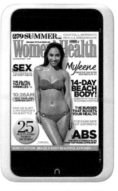

DIGITAL EDITIONS Wherever you are you can be certain you'll be able to enjoy the latest edition of your favourite magazine

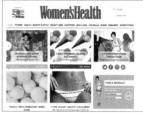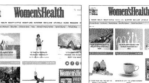

WEBSITE womenshealthmag.co.uk – fitness, health, beauty, style and more

Women'sHealth

JOIN THE UK'S FASTEST GROWING WOMEN'S MAGAZINE!

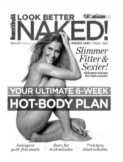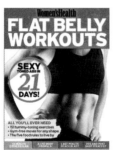

BOOKS Expert advice for all your goals

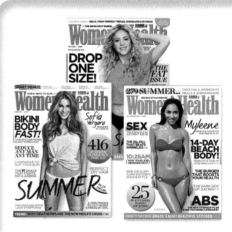

MAGAZINE Available at newsagents or by monthly subscription

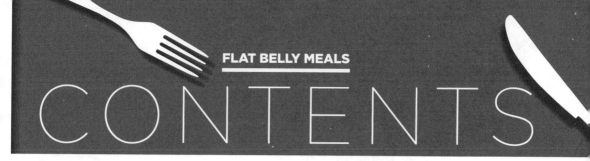

CONTENTS

*With this book you too can
get a kick-ass flat belly.
Excited? We are*

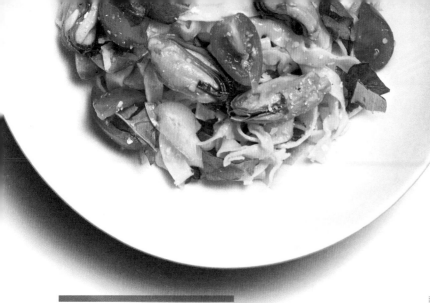

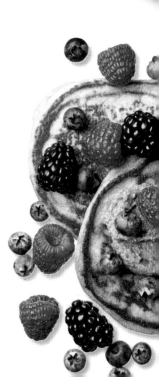

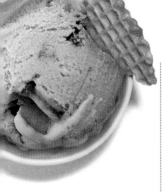

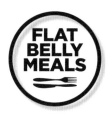

WELCOME

In the race of most-asked-about-body parts, there's only one clear winner... And since you probably clocked the title of this book before you opened it, I'm pretty sure we're both on the same page.

The Belly – the bane of so many bulge battles and a constant subject of discussion at *Women's Health* HQ. It's the most unfathomable and unfair of body parts. Studies show that for every stone you put on, more than 3lbs of it will go directly on your tummy* – a ratio that's not exactly working in your favour. And yet it's the curve you can't escape. Nobody ever asks, 'Does my belly look big in this?' Because one glimpse in the mirror at a pencil skirt pulling on a paunch or a quick glance down to see a muffin top accessorizing your new skinny jeans tells you all you need to know. It all feels so confidence-crushingly conspicuous.

This isn't just about aesthetics though. We know that abdominal fat is biologically more harmful than fat on other parts of our bodies – it promotes insulin resistance (a condition associated with type 2 diabetes) and skyrockets your chances of suffering heart disease. And bafflingly, bellies seem to exist irrespective of size, body shape or the number on the scales. I've met yoga bunnies who can plank to perfection and the sort of dedicated gym goers who actually enjoy crunches – and even they can't master the toned tummy they seemingly deserve.

So what's going on? Well, the truth is that sit-ups can only get you so far. Of course exercise is crucial (if the prone-on-the-sofa approach worked I wouldn't have a job) but it's half the story. This book is the other half. When it comes to sculpting a sexy, streamlined stomach, food matters. So from the dozens of filling, low-calorie recipes to the day-by-day balanced meal plans, the next 220 pages are packed with great, tummy-friendly food you'll actually want to make. You won't find fad diets or lose-it-quick promises; just solid, nutritionally sound suggestions that will up your energy levels and fuel your workout without widening your waist. It's a permanent way of eating.

But this book was never supposed to just be about what to eat – primarily it's about *why*. Because if there's one thing I've found, it's that *understanding* food – and fat for that matter – is the key to taking on your health demons. And this much I know... Firstly, give yourself a break. Self-hate has never helped anyone in the long run and your stomach, no matter what it looks like, deserves a little love. Belly fat *is* notoriously hard to shift (until you put this book into action, obviously), largely because women are genetically designed to store fat around the stomach and hips and not let it go easily. Getting worked up about it also makes things worse with the stress hormone cortisol sending more padding directly to your midriff.

But none of that leaves you powerless. The good news is that we're learning more about the foods that promote these processes – and of course the ones that counteract it. We know saturated fat in food isn't the enemy we once thought it was and that lower-carb diets are actually more effective at targeting stomach fat. Once you start to understand the science behind it all, food becomes an essential part of your health weaponry. It's about embracing, not avoiding. So read, create, eat, enjoy. Health never tasted so good.

Farrah Storr
Editor, Women's Health

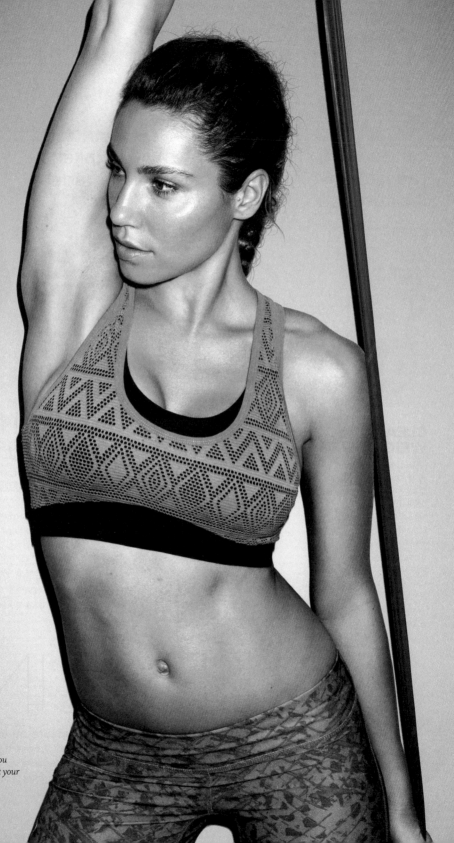

Sit-ups can only get you so far – it's time to eat your belly into submission

FIVE-SECOND FATBURNERS

Get ready to feel the burn – we've taken the latest weight-loss science and made it bite-sized, to give you a head start.

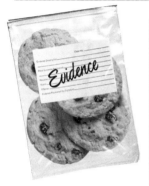

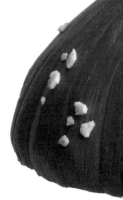

21

The average number of times that lean people chew each mouthful of their food when they're eating. This helps their bodies better digest what they've just eaten. And fatter folk? Seventeen chews. Get munching.

CLEAR UP YOUR WEIGHT GAIN

Listen up, grazers. Research in the *Journal Of Marketing* shows when food is in a clear packet, we eat up to 69% more if it's bite-sized, but up to 78% less when treats are larger. You're more likely to think one more small snack is okay, but limit yourself with larger ones, says study author Dr Xiaoyan Deng. Use clear bags for bigger snacks but opaque for bite-sized treats. Happy snacking.

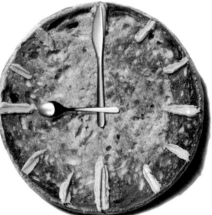

Call time on cravings

Beat morning munchies by adding peanut butter to your breakfast – you can control cravings for up to 12 hours, says a recent study*. Subjects who ate a peanut-based breakfast had higher levels of peptide YY, a hormone that makes you feel full. Buy a butter with 100% peanuts to avoid hidden calories.

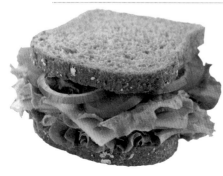

LEUCINE

An amino acid that keeps your appetite under control, helping you to feel fuller for longer. Choose turkey – which is loaded with the stuff – for your sandwiches or stir-fries if you're prone to over-gobbling. It's not just for Christmas…

PHOTOGRAPHY: GETTY, CLOCK IMAGE MARTHA PAVLIDOU FOR WEARESTUDIO33.COM. *SOURCE: BRITISH JOURNAL OF NUTRITION.

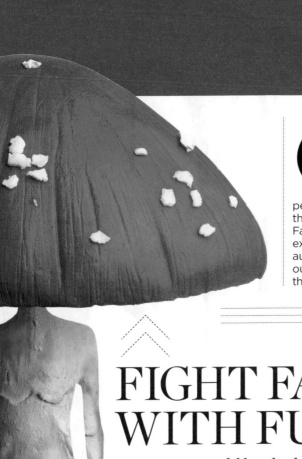

FIGHT FAT WITH FUNGI

Vitamin D could be the key to battling the bulge. Scientists at the University of Minnesota assessed athletes' body fat and found those with the lowest amount had the highest vitamin D levels. The good news is that eating just three sun-exposed mushrooms a day delivers the same amount as taking a 50mcg supplement. Place them gills-up in the sun for six hours for the biggest vit D hit. If you can't sunbathe this winter, at least your dinner can.

FLAVONOLS

Nifty chemicals which boost your metabolism for even better fat burning. And the great news is, they're found in chocolate. Just make sure it's the dark kind with over 70% cocoa – and stick to a few squares – for a beneficial choc to the system.

10

THE NUMBER OF MINUTES IT TAKES TO EVEN OUT BLOOD SUGAR WITH FENNEL. STUDIES SHOW THIS GREEN VEG'S FIBRES TRIGGER EFFECTS THAT PROTECT AGAINST OBESITY – HUNGER FADES, ENERGY IS BOOSTED AND THE LIVER SLOWS GLUCOSE PRODUCTION. TRY HALF A RAW BULB WITH LEMON JUICE TO AID DIGESTION.

SOURCE: *CELL JOURNAL*

DROWN FAT WITH COCOA

Good news: hot chocolate is healthy after all. New research shows one mug per fortnight contains enough cacao to reduce your triglyceride levels (you know, the things that spike blood sugar and insulin) and restrict fat storage*. Skip the sweetened cocoa powder though and look for a brand made with unrefined cacao instead. Vitalife Cocoa Powder (£3.49, vitalifehealth.com) is a good option. Try it with coconut milk and you've got a Bounty in a mug.

PINOLENIC ACID

Small is beautiful. Not only do pine nuts pack a superb protein punch – great for flat belly fans and gym bunnies alike – but they also contain a fatty acid substance called pinolenic acid, which is an impressive appetite supressant. Power up your pasta by roasting the nuts and sprinkling them on dishes, or making your own pesto.

1/3

The amount by which you should cut your calorie intake to make weight loss bearable. Australian research revealed this reduction increased the production of satiety hormones and the small intestine's sensitivity to food within 12 weeks.

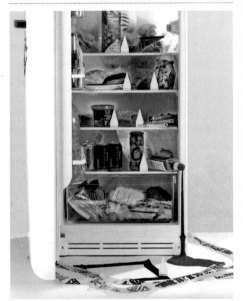

Stop the Scavenge

If you're tempted to scoff the contents of your fridge, check your watch. A study in *Obesity* showed hunger for snacks peaks at 8pm. Cheese is your best bet if you get night-time nibbles. It's practically carb-free and won't be stored as quickly by your body as fat.

GO GREEN TO CONTROL YOUR BLOOD SUGAR

Love chips? Then make a brew. Green tea could blunt the negative effects that starchy foods have on blood sugar. A study in *Molecular Nutrition And Food Research* found that mice had about half the usual increase in blood glucose when their starchy chow was spiked with a green tea compound known as EGCG. Turns out it slows the digestion of starches, leaving you feeling fuller for longer. Have a big mug of green tea with your toast in the morning and leave the bellies to the builders.

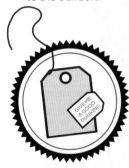

GIVE ME A GOOD DUNKING

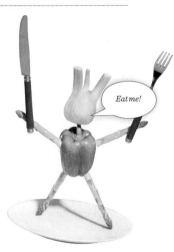

Eat me!

CUT CALORIES WITH CUTLERY

We already know smaller plates make us eat less. Now scientists from Oxford University have revealed the size and colour of cutlery is also key. In a recent study, smaller, light-coloured spoons were found to make you perceive food as sweeter and denser than if you used big dark-hued cutlery. Use a white enamel teaspoon (£10.90, clippings.com) for dessert and you'll eat away at your waistline rather than a second helping of tiramisu.

OSTEOCALCIN

A protein, found in olives and olive oil, which lets your brain know that you're not so hungry after all... Prevent a binge before it even strikes by beginning your meal with some olives, or drizzle a small amount of the oil on your food.

CONTROL CAKE RAGE

If you have a short fuse, what you eat could light it. Recent research showed those who ate more trans fats reported feeling irritable and behaving aggressively more often than those who ate less. One theory: trans fats may interfere with the production of long-chain omega-3s – fats that have been reported to reduce aggression. Don't get angry, get smart. Food manufacturers don't have to mention trans fats in their nutrition guidelines. Look out for hydrogenated or partially hydrogenated fats in the ingredients list – it means the same thing. You've been warned.

SOURCE: PLOS ONE JOURNAL

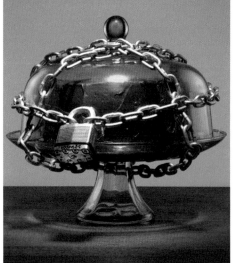

CAPSAICIN

The substance found in chillis that makes them hot in your mouth also burns off your fat. Good news if you like life fiery – chillis have been proven to curb your appetite and boost your metabolism for up to 4.5 hours. Shred a chilli in your salad dressing or sprinkle dried chillis onto your meals to boost the burn. *PHYSIOLOGY & BEHAVIOR*

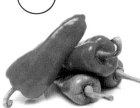

TEXT YOUR BUDDY TO TORCH MORE FAT

Turns out your iPhone is even smarter than you think. In a month-long study of dieters*, US researchers discovered a whopping 100% of those who had daily prevention texts such as "Don't overeat today" or "Stay away from the crisps at lunch", sent to their phones sustained their weight loss.

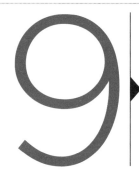

9

THE APPROXIMATE NUMBER OF POUNDS LESS THAT WOMEN WHO READ THEIR FOOD LABELS WEIGH. TRY THE CALORIE COUNTER AND TRAFFIC LIGHT FOOD CHECK APP. THE PRODUCT DATABASE HAS A THREE-COLOUR NUTRITION GUIDE, SO YOU CAN SEE IF FOODS ARE GOOD TO GO, OR SIMPLY A "NO GO".
SOURCE: *AGRICULTURAL ECONOMICS*

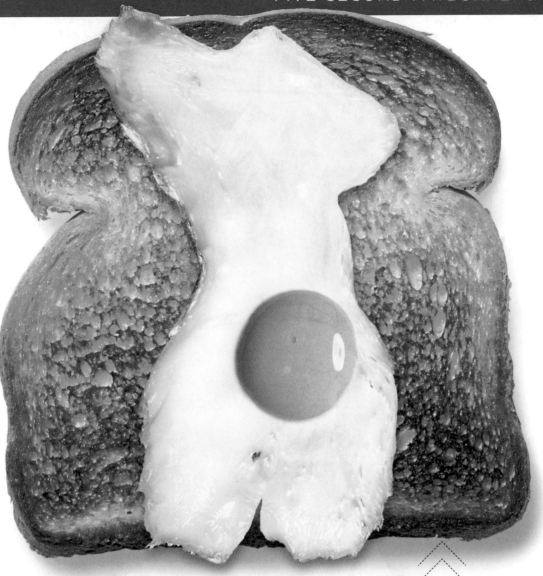

TOAST YOUR BULGE

Breakfast dodgers beware: a recent study published in the journal *Obesity* revealed that women who ate a 700-calorie breakfast and 200-calorie dinner lost more than twice as much weight over 12 weeks than those whose meal sizes were reversed. Hormone dips rev up your metabolism in the morning and make it sluggish at night, explains study author Dr Daniela Jakubowicz.

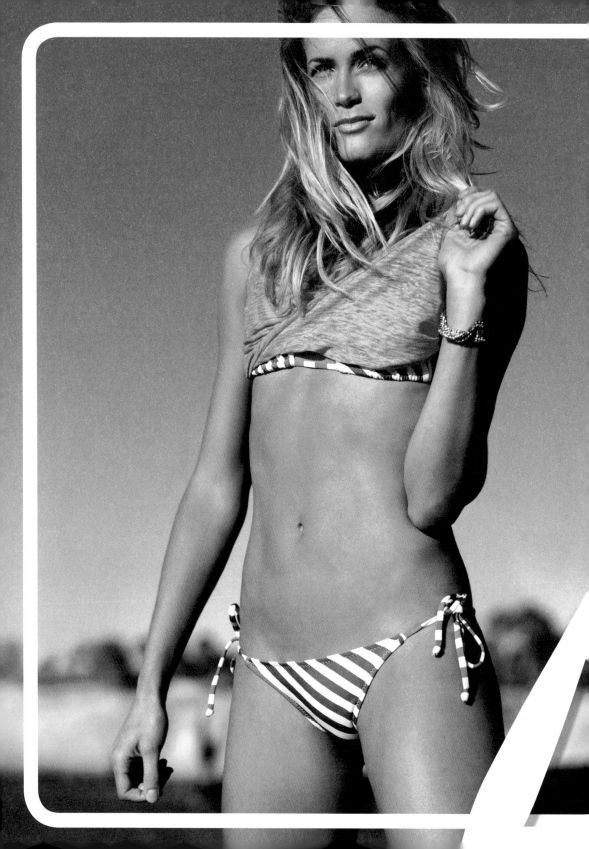

CHAPTER 1

THE
BASICS

Eating the food that slims you down
and shapes you up is easier than you
think – once you learn what different foods
do for, and against, your body. Ditch the
flimsy fad diets and read on to discover the
flat belly science behind our regime of
staying full, enjoying food, losing weight –
and keeping it off for good. *Bon appetit!*

Lose weight – not your mind

You can shed pounds without losing your marbles with these flat belly strategies

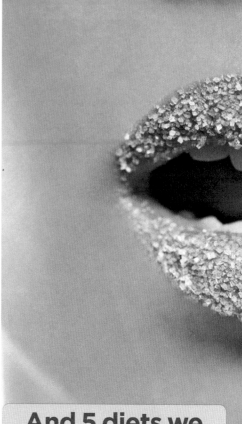

Were weight loss to come in a pill, the list of side effects would include "Causes shortness of cash" and "Users may experience a loss of friends." The trick is to make healthy eating fit your lifestyle – not the other way round. Follow these new rules for lasting results, with none of the unpleasant extras.

1 MAKE IT WALLET-FRIENDLY

Forty two per cent of Brits say they'd eat better if healthy food was cheaper, according to a Food Standards Agency survey. One easy cash-saving tactic is to eat less meat. Not only is it pricey, it's a source of excess calories and saturated fat, says registered dietitian Dawn Jackson Blatner. Get your five-a-day on the cheap in the freezer aisle: frozen veg often packs more nutrients than fresh. And always cook them straight from the freezer – studies show they'll retain more vitamin C than if you let them thaw first.

2 EAT YOURSELF HAPPY

Drastically cutting calories causes your levels of the feel-good hormone serotonin to nosedive. "Unbalanced meals can also cause massive

And 5 diets we won't be trying

Weight-loss ideas to consign to life's WTF bin

THE TAPEWORM "DIET"
Pop a pill containing a tapeworm egg, then play host to a parasite that'll feed off your stomach contents.
Side-effects There's a worm inside you. Also, there's a slight chance of death.

"VISION-DIET" GLASSES
These Japanese-invented specs have a blue tint that makes your food look unappetising.
Side-effects Eating out isn't as much fun. And you'll look like Bono.

THE HALLELUJAH
You can only eat the foods mentioned in Genesis Chapter 1, Verse 29.
Side effects It's an 85 per cent raw diet. It's going to be tedious.

"SMALL-BITE" FALSE TEETH
Wear these during meals and you'll only be able to take tiny bites of food.
Side effects You're wearing false teeth.

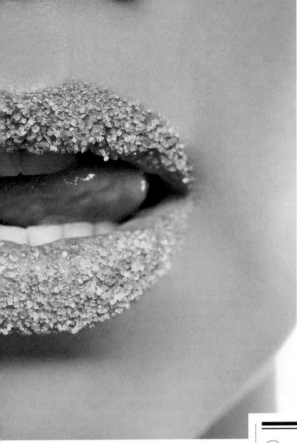

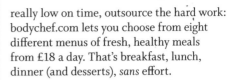

really low on time, outsource the hard work: bodychef.com lets you choose from eight different menus of fresh, healthy meals from £18 a day. That's breakfast, lunch, dinner (and desserts), *sans* effort.

4 MUSCLE UP

To keep your metabolism humming, lift weights. Muscle burns up to nine times more calories than fat, says personal trainer and weight-loss management specialist Laura Williams. She advises weight training three times a week to maintain muscle mass. The best exercises to do: squats, lunges, deadlifts and press-ups. "These recruit multiple muscle groups so they're time-efficient," Williams says. And to help that muscle repair faster, try to eat around 130g of protein a day. The morning is the optimum time to replenish protein stores, so aim for a 30g serving (that's two eggs and three tablespoons of ricotta).

fluctuations in blood sugar levels, leading to dips in energy and mood," says Nigel Denby, spokesman from the British Dietetic Association. Instead of starving yourself, switch to smarter foods. Omega-3 fatty acids (found in salmon, mackerel and eggs, amongst others) are proven mood boosters and can stabilise blood sugar. Give yourself an easy blast of omega-3 by sprinkling a tablespoon of flaxseeds over cereal, and have a tuna sandwich for lunch.

3 SCHEDULE IN SHOPPING

Not having enough time is the main barrier for 27 per cent of you, says Britain's National Obesity Observatory. But taking an hour to plan a week's worth of meals will pay off, big time. To help, download the app Menu Planner (£1.99), which plans your meals, downloads your favourite healthy recipes and tracks what you've got in your pantry. If you're

Get your five-a-day on the cheap in the freezer aisle: frozen veg often packs more nutrients than fresh.

5 ENJOY A NIGHT OUT

Trying to ditch a few pounds should never turn you into a recluse. You just have to be smart. Download the free Restaurant Nutrition app, which lists most UK restaurants and tells you how many grammes of fat really do lurk in that hot chicken salad. Better still try Weight Loss Sensei (BlackBerry, £1.50). It asks behavioural psychologists to devise eating plans that fit your lifestyle.

Your 24/7 fat burn

Morning jog or 7pm spin class? Porridge before the gym or after?
Here are the timing secrets to torching fat

7AM
DOWN HALF A PINT

As soon your alarm blares, down 500ml cold water. A German study found it boosts metabolism by 24 per cent for 90 minutes because your body must spend extra energy to bring the cold water down to your core temperature. Pop a bottle in the fridge before you go to bed so it's ready for you when you wake up.

7:30AM
BURN BEFORE BREKKIE

You can burn nearly 20 per cent more fat if you work out before you eat your porridge, says a study in the British Journal Of Nutrition. "Your blood-sugar levels are low, so your body has to use fat as fuel for your muscles to work," says Dean Hodgkin, international fat loss and fitness expert. Gym it on an empty stomach then.

8:45AM
TUCK INTO A STEAK

It might turn your stomach, but research in the British Journal Of Nutrition found eating high-protein meals such as red meat and nuts at breakfast led to a greater feeling of fullness. Try a turkey breast, one of the leanest meats, and a handful of almonds – a great source of monounsaturated fat that helps burn belly fat.

12:30PM
LOAD UP ON LUNCH

A study in the International Journal Of Obesity found those who ate 40 per cent of their daily calories from carbs and protein before 3pm dropped an average of 11 per cent of their body weight, compared with nine per cent among those who ate their big meal at dinner. Try a fist-sized baked sweet potato with chilli con carne.

12:35PM
POP A PROBIOTIC

According to a study in the European Journal Of Clinical Nutrition, taking the probiotic lactobacillus gasseri for 12 weeks reduced belly fat by a total of 4.6 per cent. Taking it mid-meal will "boost

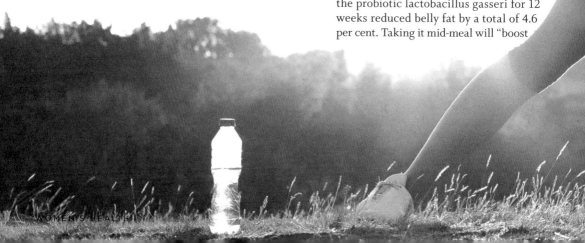

satiety and the feeling of fullness," says nutritionist Carrie Ruxton. Try Probio-Intensive, (£7.29 for 30 capsules, highernature.co.uk).

4PM
HAVE A BREW
Green tea is rich in a plant compound called ECGC, which promotes fat burning. In fact, three cups a day could cut your weight by nearly five per cent, says a French study. Go for matcha green tea powder – it can increase the body's rate of calorie burn by up to 40 per cent*. Try Clearspring Organic Matcha, (£9.99, clearspring.co.uk).

6:45PM
CHOW DOWN EARLY
To maximise weight loss, eat dinner early, then fast for around 14 hours

until breakfast the next day. Try a lean protein such as chicken or fish with green vegetables sautéed with red chilli flakes. It will raise your metabolism for the three hours after you eat, helping to burn the calories eaten during the day.

8PM
WALK IT OFF
You've had dinner, now go for a 10-minute walk. Light post-meal exercise can lower blood sugar and stop you storing fat*. If it's too cold to venture out, try this yoga pose, known to relieve indigestion: lie with your hands on your knees, exhale and hug your knees to your chest. Rock from side to side for five to 10 breaths.

11PM
GET SOME SHUT-EYE
Poor sleepers are more likely to suffer major weight gain*, so aim for seven hours to keep cortisol levels in check. "This hormone regulates appetite," says personal trainer Christianne Wolff. "If it is out of sync you'll never feel full." And probably won't fit six watches on your wrist, either.

You can burn nearly 20% more fat if you work out before you eat your porridge

Swot up, slim down

Getting in shape requires a bit of maths, genetics, psychology and physiology.
What's your weight-loss formula? Take our quiz to find out

1
All calories are...

A EQUAL ☑
B NOT EQUAL ☑

2
Match the food item to the correct portion size:

CHEESE	GOLF BALL
PEANUT BUTTER	TENNIS BALL
FISH	HOCKEY PUCK
RICE, PASTA OR PRETZELS	CHEQUE BOOK
BAGEL	MATCH BOX
CHOCOLATE	TENNIS BALL
ICE CREAM	DOMINO

3
Once you reach your goal weight...

A YOU CAN SHORTEN YOUR WORKOUTS ☑
B JUST GO BACK TO EATING NORMALLY ☑
C YOU'LL ALWAYS HAVE TO EAT A BIT LESS ☑
D YOU'LL BE NATURALLY AND BIOLOGICALLY 'SLIM' ☑

4
IF YOU HAVE FAT PARENTS...

A YOU'RE DOOMED, SO CRY ☑
B IT DOESN'T MATTER – YOU'RE IN CHARGE OF YOUR OWN METABOLISM ☑
C YES, YOU'RE MORE PRONE TO PACKING ON EXTRA POUNDS, BUT YOU'RE STILL IN CONTROL OF YOUR HEALTH ☑
D YOU SHOULD BE TESTED TO FIND OUT IF YOU CARRY THE FAT GENE ☑

5
Your willpower...

A IS LOCKED SOMEWHERE BETWEEN YOUR LOVE OF MINI EGGS AND MAGNUM PISTACHIOS ☑
B EBBS AND FLOWS, BASED ON YOUR ENVIRONMENT ☑
C STRENGTHENS WITH TRAINING, LIKE A MUSCLE ☑
D DOESN'T ACTUALLY AFFECT YOUR WEIGHT LOSS ☑

6
Circle the picture(s) of the best after-workout recovery food(s):

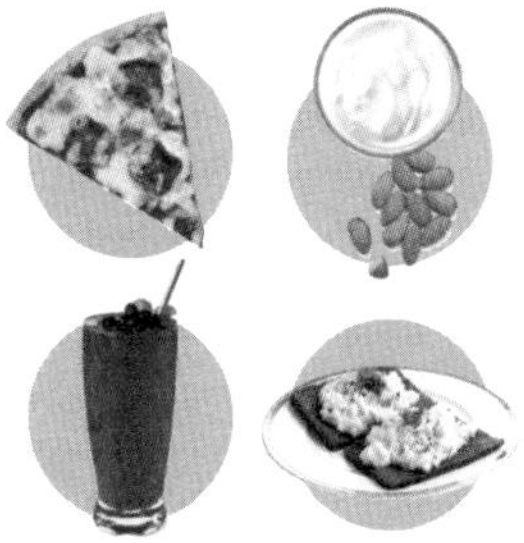

7
Switching to diet drinks...

A MAKES THIS WHOLE WEIGHT-LOSS THING A BREEZE ☑
B WILL KEEP YOU FULL ☑
C MEANS THE FOOD MARKETERS WON ☑
D CURBS YOUR SUGAR CRAVINGS ☑

8
Gluten free...

A IS BETTER FOR EVERYONE ☑
B IS A PAINLESS WAY TO CUT CALORIES ☑
C WON'T BLOAT YOU ☑
D CAN HAVE MORE ADDITIVES THAN REGULAR PRODUCTS ☑

WORDS: ANITA BHAGWANDAS AND CINDY KUZMA

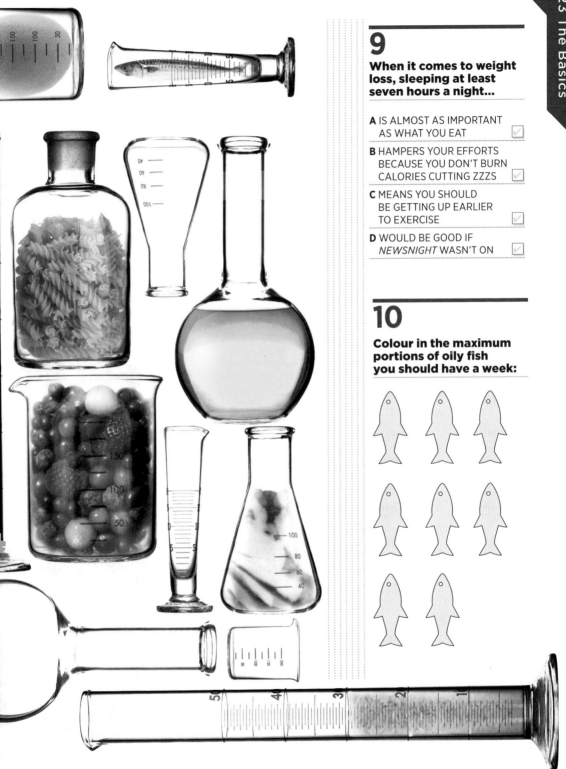

9

When it comes to weight loss, sleeping at least seven hours a night...

A IS ALMOST AS IMPORTANT AS WHAT YOU EAT ☑

B HAMPERS YOUR EFFORTS BECAUSE YOU DON'T BURN CALORIES CUTTING ZZZS ☑

C MEANS YOU SHOULD BE GETTING UP EARLIER TO EXERCISE ☑

D WOULD BE GOOD IF *NEWSNIGHT* WASN'T ON ☑

10

Colour in the maximum portions of oily fish you should have a week:

ANSWER 1

B

As a unit of energy output from a certain food type, a calorie is a calorie, says nutritionist and dietitian Hala El-Shafie. But our macronutrients (carbs, fats and protein) serve different functions, and their calories are used differently in the body. For example, protein requires the most energy to burn and keeps you feeling full longer.

> YOUR MOVE

To gauge your daily calorie needs, take your target weight, multiply it by your weekly training hours and add a number from 9 to 11 (representing the intensity of your workouts). Make sure the result includes a gram of protein per pound of your goal weight.

ANSWER 2

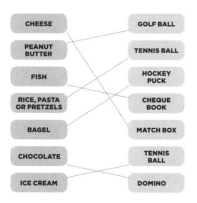

CHEESE	GOLF BALL
PEANUT BUTTER	TENNIS BALL
FISH	HOCKEY PUCK
RICE, PASTA OR PRETZELS	CHEQUE BOOK
BAGEL	MATCH BOX
CHOCOLATE	TENNIS BALL
ICE CREAM	DOMINO

> YOUR MOVE

Forget measuring every morsel, just keep the equivalent object in mind when dishing up. Be vigilant when tired – studies show that's when people up portion sizes. To avoid serving too much, start a photo diary. But don't tweet it – nobody wants to be that person.

ANSWER 3

C

Maintaining your goal weight takes as much effort as the initial loss. The new, leaner you requires 300 fewer calories a day, according to a study at Columbia University in New York. For an easy maintenance strategy, simply cut out the carbohydrates from one of your daily meals. Hasta la vista, pasta.

> YOUR MOVE

People who work out for at least 30 minutes a day are more successful at keeping fat away, according to the journal *Clinical Nutrition*. And you can bring your chocolate to the gym. "Eat treats after you work out so the calories are used for fuel, not stored as fat," says WHPT Anwar Gilbert.

ANSWER 4

C

Scientists have identified several obesity genes, including FTO, a single variation of which can raise your obesity odds by up to 30 per cent. Still, "While genetic factors play a role in obesity, they don't prevent weight loss," says Dr Robert Ziltzer, of the Scottsdale Weight Loss Center in Arizona, US.

> YOUR MOVE

Don't bother with an FTO test. At worst it will sap your motivation. In a study, adults with a fat-promoting copy of FTO reduced its effects by 30 per cent with just an hour's exercise a week. Make it your goal to work out daily and you'll negate your fat genes – stat.

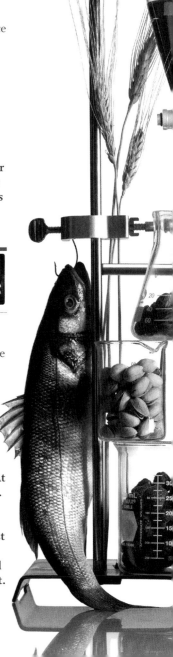

ANSWER 5

B&C

"Willpower isn't constant – it goes up and down based on your environment," explains Dr Sherry Pagoto, a clinical psychology professor at the University of Massachusetts. Spend a dull meeting staring at a pile of doughnuts, and you'll end up with sugar on your face, but remove temptation from the picture and you'll resist dessert like a total pro. Simple enough.

> **YOUR MOVE**
Feeling stressed leads to bad choices, so sugary snacks start to look extremely tempting when you're still at your desk at 9pm. Instead, have a Green & Black's mini Maya Gold bar.

ANSWER 6

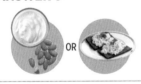

Thanks to all its fruit, that giant smoothie may harbour twice the number of calories you just burned. So pick Greek yoghurt and nuts or eggs on rye. Protein-rich recovery foods replenish your glycogen stores and give you the raw materials you need to build new muscle.

> **YOUR MOVE**
A recent study found protein with a little carbs is best. Still fancy a shake? Get the perfect ratio with this one, within 20 minutes of working out: half a banana, protein powder, almond milk and flaxseed.

ANSWER 7

C

According to a US study, artificial sweeteners in diet drinks may stave off sweet cravings – but, says lead researcher Susan Swithers, "You've messed up the system, so when you consume real sugar, your body doesn't know if it should process it because it's been tricked before."

> **YOUR MOVE**
Want the bubbles without the sugar-brain trickery? Opt for sparkling water with a few slices of lemon, lime or cucumber for added flavour and vitamins. Often, it's just the fizziness we crave in drinks, not the taste of sugar.

ANSWER 8

 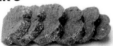

D

It's a common misconception that gluten-free means good for you. Warburton's Free From sliced white bread has 2.2g fat per slice and 80 calories, compared with 0.5g per slice and 58 calories in its regular loaf. Before you buy, check the labels of food products, so you don't get caught out.

> **YOUR MOVE**
Dr Sarah Brewer says: "Rye bread, which contains significantly less gluten than wheat bread, helps to suppress hunger. Have it at breakfast to reduce your appetite until lunch and this effect will continue into the afternoon, curbing your cravings."

ANSWER 9

A

A study in *Annals Of Internal Medicine* suggests people who sleep 5.5 hours may burn 400 fewer calories the next day than those who get 8.5 hours. Scientists believe this is due to increases in the hunger hormone ghrelin and dips in the satiety hormone leptin that occur when we're tired.

> **YOUR MOVE**
To get a decent night's sleep, turn off the TV (or Netflix) at least 90 minutes before bed. That goes for your smartphone, too, as studies show that the blue glow the screen emits can suppress sleep hormone melatonin.

ANSWER 10

If you're pregnant, breastfeeding, or planning to have kids at some point, stick to two portions of fish a week. Oily types (like salmon, mackerel and sardines) can contain polychlorinated biphenyls – a type of pollutant that won't have an immediate effect on your health but can build up over time to impair your reproductive system.

> **YOUR MOVE**
Look for a supplement with choline, a compound that helps to metabolise lipids. Try The Omega 3, which you can buy at Tom Oliver Nutrition.

PHOTOGRAPHY: GALLERY STOCK, GETTY IMAGES. TOM OLIVER NUTRITION THE OMEGA 3 (£39.99, TOMOLIVERNUTRITION.COM)

Can you count on calories?

If you've been counting calories all this time, stop now! These two plates might feature the same numbers, but nutritionist Zoë Harcombe is here to explain how one is the secret to eating more and weighing less

'A calorie is a calorie' (and all calories are evil horrible things) is the grand maxim upon which the multi-billion dieting industry is based. Consume less, expend more energy and thou shalt lose weight. It all sounds sensible, right? Wrong.

Mounting research shows we've been fed a big fat lie. Calorie counting is not the answer for either short-term or long-term weight loss. The real solution lies in turning around the ratio of carbohydrates to protein and fat in our diets, and harnessing the power of the way our bodies metabolise calories once they enter our system. What does this mean? Put quite simply, you will be able to eat the same, if not more, than you used to but effectively consume 200 fewer calories a day.

We know calories are not equal nutritionally – 100 calories of table sugar has no essential fats, no protein, no vitamins and no minerals, while 100 calories of liver (I know – me neither) provides virtually every nutrient that a human needs, even if it doesn't taste quite so good in cakes. But

> Trying to cut calories often leads us to make the wrong food choices

calories are also not equal metabolically. You see, the minute we put calories into our body, they behave in very different ways. I'm going to show how you can make sure the ones you eat behave themselves properly.

Surprisingly, the problem with counting calories begins before you've even put them in your mouth. Weight gain can begin as early as in the supermarket aisle because trying to cut calories often leads us to make entirely the wrong food choices.

With four calories for approximately every gram of carbohydrate compared with nine calories per gram of fat, we've learned to shun fat in favour of carbs. But it's actually those fat calories that are the ones most likely to be used up by the body's own personal command centre – otherwise known as the basal metabolic rate (BMR).

Forget diamonds, the BMR is a girl's best friend. It's the system that means you burn calories even when you're lying in bed. Even inactive, your body has a shed load to do just to keep you alive, powering the nine systems in the body (skeletal, nervous, endocrine, digestive, respiratory, circulatory, lymphatic, urinary and reproductive).

The taller, heavier and younger we are, the more work the body has to do and the higher our basal metabolic rate. Contrary to popular belief, dieting isn't about starving the BMR of the calories it needs, it's about

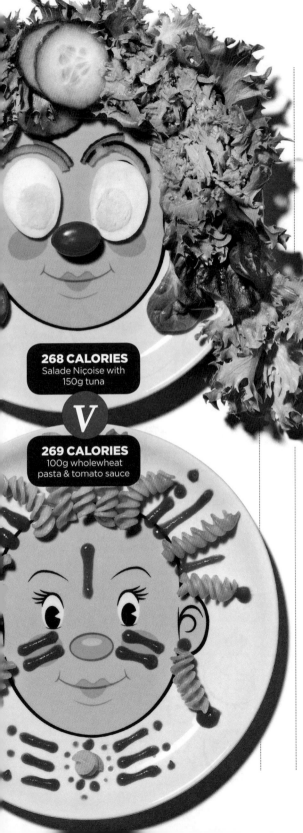

268 CALORIES
Salade Niçoise with
150g tuna

V

269 CALORIES
100g wholewheat
pasta & tomato sauce

providing your body with the right number of calories it can most easily metabolise. Just like with men it's the quality, *not* the quantity, that counts. The trick is not to think about total calories, but to think separately about the calories you need for body maintenance and those needed for energy. For example: if you're around 5ft 6in, 9ish stone and in your late twenties, your BMR is approximately 1,400 calories (the number your body needs to run itself).

In your late thirties, your metabolism slows and your BMR drops to 1,360 calories and in your late forties it's around 1,320. That means if you exercise regularly, you will need around 775 calories on top of your body repair needs. These are the calories needed to meet the body's energy requirements. But, contrary to what we've previously been told, carbohydrates are not the only way to get this energy. The time has come to start thinking about fuelling your body from fat.

FAT'S THE ANSWER

While we've been busying ourselves putting our maths skills to good use by counting calories, we haven't been thinking about what our body actually does with them the minute they enter our digestive system.

If you paid attention in biology class, you might remember that carbs are for energy. Which is true – but that's all they're for. It turns out that only fat and protein can help with those BMR jobs – and that any carbohydrate that you eat is useless for repair work. Visualise a little operations manager sitting within your body with a check-list of things to do every day: pump the heart, work the liver, filter the kidneys, repair cells etc.

Every time fat, protein, vitamins and minerals come in, the ops manager can direct those nutrients to things on the to-do list; but every time carbs report for duty, nothing gets crossed off the list. That's why professional cyclists have been known to carry around pats of butter with them to keep them going through a long race.

If you don't fancy putting a pack of Lurpak in your gym bag, opt for some oily fish or red meat rather than brown rice and vegetables. Not only will you have valuable fuel to supercharge your workouts, you'll also have the fat and protein needed to repair the cells you're about to push to the limit.

Dr Barry Groves, author of *Trick And Treat: How 'Healthy Eating' Is Making Us Ill*, says, "Only excess carbohydrates are converted to body fats; dietary proteins and fats have other essential jobs to do. Their calories are not stored and don't count." So that rare porterhouse steak, cooked in butter, could be your ticket to better and more sustainable health. Doesn't that sound delicious?

CALORIES BURN CALORIES

Your body uses up a certain number of calories breaking down whatever you eat. The efficiency of this process differs between macronutrients – that's carbs, fat, protein and, of all of them, protein requires the most calories to be properly digested.

A study from the University of Lausanne showed that only approximately 6-8 per cent of the carbohydrate calories we eat are used up in converting that carbohydrate into energy, compared with a whopping 25-30 per cent to metabolise protein. Healthy eating is less about counting calories, then, and

YOUR BEST LUNCH OPTION

Salade Niçoise has zero carb calories – its energy is used to fuel the body's systems

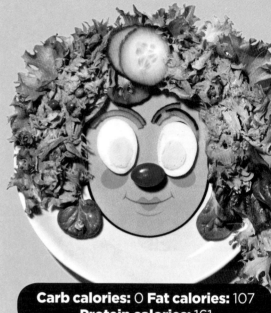

Carb calories: 0 Fat calories: 107 Protein calories: 161

VS WHOLEWHEAT PASTA AND TOMATO SAUCE: CARB CALORIES: **188**; FAT CALORIES: **45**; PROTEIN CALORIES: **36**

A TALE OF TWO MEALS

Even dishes that look and sound healthy can be secret calorie traps. Here's our guide to the dos and don'ts of everyday eating

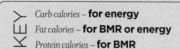

KEY
Carb calories – **for energy**
Fat calories – **for BMR or energy**
Protein calories – **for BMR**

BREAKFAST (400 CALORIES)
2 eggs (poached) on 1 slice rye bread + butter VS 2 thick slices brown toast with a banana. The egg meal has eight times as many fat calories, but 75% of the toast meal will be stored as fat

WINNER
Carb calories – 296
Fat calories – 36
Protein calories – 68
TOTAL CALORIES: 400

VS

LOSER
Carb calories – 57
Fat calories – 281
Protein calories – 62
TOTAL CALORIES: 400

more about looking at the ratio in which we consume those calories. For example, if an average woman's 2,175 calories are consumed in the 55:30:15 carb:fat:protein ratio that is currently recommended by the government, 1,986 calories are available to the body. If the same 2,175 calories were consumed in a 15:30:55 high-protein diet, (keeping fat exactly the same and swapping carbs out and protein in), the calories available to the body drops to 1,806 and, on top of that, these calories are the ones most readily used up by the body's daily needs, meaning less weight gain for you and less time needed to be spent on the cross trainer.

Let's compare two women – one only eats the real food that the planet provides – we're talking meat, eggs and dairy, fish, nuts, seeds, vegetables and fruit. The other follows public health dietary advice, making more than half her meals carb-based.If you flip the carb and protein allocations around (not because macronutrient targets are good, but because it will help to illustrate the difference that upping your protein and fat consumption can make to your body's bottom line) to the ratios above, Ms Government Advice ends up with 300 extra calories of the wrong macronutrients, leaving her short of the fat and protein calories required for her body's maintenance.

Interestingly, even with 100 calories left over from fat/protein, Ms Real Food was short by just under 400 calories for her energy needs. As a result, her body will have to break

down triglycerides (i.e. burn body fat), to keep her going, creating the perfect conditions for optimum weight loss. Ms Government Advice, on the other hand, has more than 300 extra carbohydrate calories which are likely to be stored as fat rather than them being burnt off, which of course will do nothing to aid her weight-loss. All in all, the real food diet beats everything we've been told before. So, the next time you overhear someone at your local supermarket saying 'a calorie is a calorie', you can simply smile knowingly to yourself, then head home

Your body uses a certain amount of calories to break down whatever you eat

to tuck into your cheese omelette cooked in butter, safe in the knowledge that your clever body is poised to burn those remaining calories right off. What could be more delicious than that? **WH**

Zoë Harcombe is the author of *Stop Counting Calories & Start Losing Weight* (£9.99, Columbus Publishing Limited). Fred and Friends Ms Food Face Plate, £12.50, John Lewis

---

LUNCH (325-350 CALORIES)
Pret Italian Chicken Salad VS Pret Deluxe Bento Box
90% of the chicken salad can be used for repair, but less than half of the bento box can

WINNER

Carb calories – 31
Fat calories – 206
Protein calories – 87

TOTAL CALORIES: 324

VS

LOSER

Carb calories – 200
Fat calories – 901
Protein calories – 65

TOTAL CALORIES: 355

DINNER (414 CALORIES)
280g steak with a few wedges of sweet potatoes VS 140g steak with a large baked potato. Go heavy on steak and light on chips and the 'repair' calories double, as energy calories plummet

WINNER

Carb calories – 42
Fat calories – 158
Protein calories – 241

TOTAL CALORIES: 414

VS

LOSER

Carb calories – 210
Fat calories – 79
Protein calories – 125

TOTAL CALORIES: 414

20 Smarter ways to eat

Science-heavy nutritional information can be hard to digest. Instead, knock back this bite-sized advice from the world's leading experts

1 Eat the rainbow. No, really.
"I always ask 'Where are the colours?' when I look at a plate," says dietitian Ellie Krieger. "There should be a full spectrum to get different antioxidants." For example, red peppers contain twice as much metabolism-supporting vitamin C as green.

2 Bake a much better cake
"Angel food cake is a great low-cal alternative, with no egg yolks or butter," says dietitian and BDA spokesperson Judy Watermeyer. Get tips at videojug.com/film – or pick up a packet mix (£3.59, americansweets.co.uk).

3 Freeze for better snacks
Don't toss brown bananas – freeze them and use in baking. "If you get the nibbles when watching TV, a frozen banana makes a healthy alternative to ice cream," says dietitan and BDA spokesperson Melissa Rice. Cool.

4 Double up for more iron
Too tired to give your all at the gym? You probably need to top up your iron supplies. "Vitamin C helps our body absorb iron from our food. Try drinking a glass of orange juice with cereal or have tomatoes with steak," says dietitian Kelly McCabe. Try vine-ripened tomatoes if you can – store them in a fruit bowl, though, as the fridge impairs their flavour.

5 Scale down every meal
"Stop before you're full and still want to eat more," says Krieger. "Not in a negative, deprived way – but on a scale of 1 to 10, if 10 is Christmas-full and you usually eat till you're at 8, try stopping at 6. You'll feel and look better."

6 Up your omegas-3s
"For an easy way to increase the amount of fibre and omega-3 fatty acids in your diet, sprinkle ground flaxseed over cereal and salads," says Pippa Kendrick, author of *The Intolerant Gourmet* (£20, HarperCollins). "You can even bake with it – add 2 tbsp flaxseed mixed with 3 tbsp water instead of an egg."

7 Boost the burn with spices
Spices don't just deliver a kick to your tastebuds – they'll give your metabolism a boot up the backside too. Food scientist Heidi Allison, author of *The Chili Pepper Diet*, found that you can lose 10 times as much weight if you add a sprinkle of dried chillies to your meals. Meanwhile, the polyphenols in cinnamon are amazing at regulating insulin, heading off those blood sugar spikes that lead to cravings. Sprinkle some on your latte or mix it in with your bowl of porridge at breakfast for a natural sweetener. Spice up your life.

You can lose 10 times
as much weight if
you add a sprinkle
of dried chillies
to your meals

*When it comes
to cutting calories,
everyone loves
a good squeeze*

8 Cut calories with lemons

"Lemon is my secret weapon," says chef Katie Lee, author of *The Comfort Table*. "Squeeze the juice or sprinkle the zest over vegetables instead of using extra oil or butter. You can sauté spinach with just a teaspoon of oil, and add lemon juice for a lot of flavour without all the calories."

9 Shrink your tableware

"Buy smaller, more delicate dinner plates," says Sally Bee, author of *Have Your Cake and Eat it Too* (£14.99, HarperCollins). "Your portion sizes will drop, followed by your waistline." For main meals, a plate with a 10-inch diameter is ideal, or try the Healthy Portion Plate (£8.99, amazon.co.uk) for a visual guide.

10 Get scribbling

Write down everything you eat and drink – at the time you're scoffing it down – for one week. "If you see 'four biscuits' on your list it may make you think twice before taking a fifth!" says dietitian Natalie Jones. Try using the Food Diary app (£1.99, itunes).

11 Snack smart with eggs

"Eggs have only 70 calories and provide protein, vitamin D, iron and omega-3s," says sports dietitian Leslie Bonci. Boil an egg and chop onto an oat cracker for a tasty snack with hit of zinc and omega-3s. Tasty and nutritious!

12 Walk on the wild side

"Unusual foods tend to be healthier because they're raised or grown in nature," says food author Stephen Perrine. For a body-friendly change try choosing venison over beef, pheasant over chicken or watercress over lettuce.

13 Eat like it's Monday

"Think of each meal as a clean slate, an individual opportunity to eat well," says Glassman. "If you've been eating a lot of fried foods or sweets, don't throw in the towel and have more — start fresh every time you eat."

14 Make pasta healthier

"Adding a little vinegar to starchy food lowers its glycaemic index," says dietitian Rene Smalberger. Toss wholewheat pasta with olive oil and 2 tbsps balsamic to slow down the burn and keep hunger at bay.

> Research found that if you eat listening to music, you'll consume 450 more calories

15 Stay young with seeds

"Sesame seeds are high in copper, which research in the *American Journal of Clinical Nutrition* found can reduce grey hairs," says nutritionist Natalie McAdam. Sprinkle them into stir-fries and use tahini – sesame seed paste – as a sandwich spread.

16 Relax and then eat

"It's better for your physiological and psychological health to savour your meal," says dietitian Evelyn Tribole. And turn off your iPod, too. Research found that if you eat listening to music you'll consume 450 more calories.

17 Add heat to eat less

"Hot food is more satiating, so you'll eat less of it," says dietitian Dawn Jackson

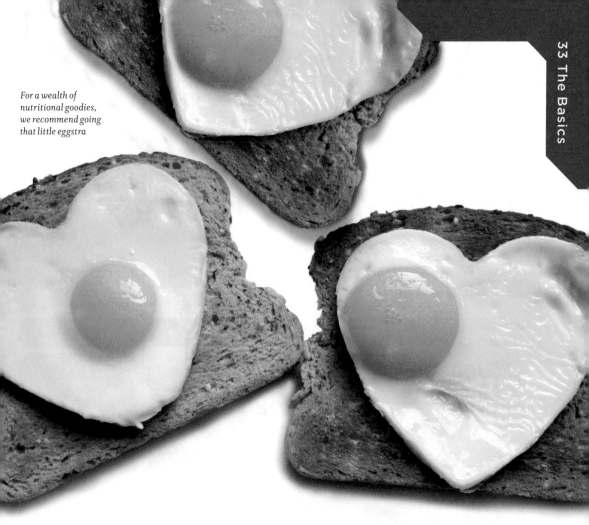

For a wealth of nutritional goodies, we recommend going that little eggstra

Blatner. Take an extra minute to zap that leftover pizza in the microwave or add something warm like chicken or grilled halloumi to a salad.

18 Give peas a chance
"Get an extra portion of veggies with a handful of frozen peas," says dietitian and BDA spokesperson Dr Frankie Phillips. "Eat from the freezer – refreshing, nutritious and surprisingly tasty!"

19 Go for the orange
No, we're not talking about fake tan. "Swap your regular potatoes at dinner for sweet potatoes – they're higher in vitamins and minerals and have a lower GI to help stabilise blood sugar," says McCabe. You don't even have to miss out on chips – use an Airfryer (£204.25, phillips.co.uk) to make sweet potato fries and you'll knock off 80 per cent of the fat of your usual treat. That sounds pretty tasty to us!

20 Ditch the gimmicks
"Beware of those diets that promise results through elimination of entire food groups," says Dr Jennifer Anderson, a professor of food science at Colorado State University. "Crazy rules like 'Eat fruit only in the morning' are gimmicks." Good, we weren't sold on the idea of having to empty our well-stocked cupboards WH

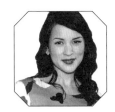

MY FLAT BELLY DIARY:

Rachel Khoo

Paris-based TV star chef Rachel Khoo is a firm believer in
the French diet – her cross-channel slimming tips are all gain and no pain

MONDAY

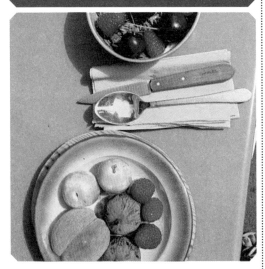

8am
*Muesli with a fruit plate
and orange juice*

11am
Herbal tea and an apple

1pm
*Salmon with potato gratis
and spinach*

3pm
Chamomile tea

7:30pm
*Cheese ravioli with tomato
sauce and olives*

I've been away
from home, filming
in Europe, this week.
I always steer clear
of desserts when
I'm on the road as
I can't exercise
to balance it out. It's
important that I stay
aware of what I'm
eating, especially
when I have to taste
so many dishes
when I'm on set.

TUESDAY

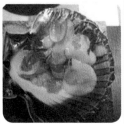

9am
*Muesli with yoghurt, berries
and a green tea*

10:30am
*Sparkling water
and a banana*

1:30pm
Fish with mushrooms.

4pm
Ginger tea

8pm
*Swedish tapas with venison,
ravioli and smoked salmon*

I love the small-plate
culture in Europe.
It's great for travelling
because you can
sample a lot of dishes
but you don't feel
as if you're going
to roll out of the
restaurant afterwards.

WEDNESDAY

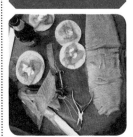

8:30am
*Muesli with yoghurt, berries
and a green tea*

11am
Mint tea

2pm
*Smoked salmon on
rye crackers*

4pm
Green tea and an apple

8pm
*Steak with vegetables
and potatoes*

When I'm in London,
I go to two hour-long
hip-hop dance classes
a week. I'm really
awful at dancing
but for me it's more
about spending the
hour with my friends
and having fun.

THURSDAY	FRIDAY	SATURDAY	SUNDAY

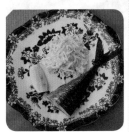

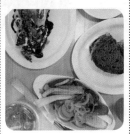

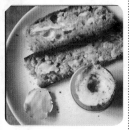

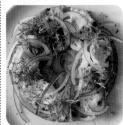

THURSDAY

4am
Fresh beetroot, apple and ginger smoothie

9am
Cup of tea and a cheese sandwich

1pm
Grilled mackerel with a salad and fizzy water

5:30pm
Tapas with ham and potato croquetas with a glass of rioja

It's really nice to unwind with a glass of wine but when I'm filming I stick to fizzy water and gallons of herbal tea. I only drink fruit juice if it's freshly pressed.

FRIDAY

9am
Muesli with yoghurt, berries and a green tea

11am
Various dishes on set (above)

2pm
Gazpacho and seafood paella

5pm
Banana and sparkling water

8pm
Fish with vegetables and a glass of wine

I love having fruit in the morning. I do like cooked breakfasts as well, but I tend to save them for a weekend treat. Muesli keeps me just full enough until lunchtime.

SATURDAY

9:30am
Boiled egg with soldiers and herbal tea

1pm
Paella with a green salad

3pm
Fresh figs

7:30pm
Tapas with ham and potato croquetas, patatas bravas, olives, cheese and flatbread with tomatoes

I've just started a class called Flywheel. It's a 60-minute session that's a bit like spinning, but they give you an upper body workout, too. I do it once or twice a week.

SUNDAY

9am
Muesli with chopped bananas and yoghurt, green tea

1pm
Fish cooked over an open fire with salad

5pm
Cheese and red onion bagel and tea with milk

9pm
Cheese and crackers

It's hard to get something nutritious when travelling, so I just grab what I can. I ate a lot of cheese today so I might try to squeeze in an extra gym class next week.

THE EXPERT VERDICT

Resident nutritionist Dr Christy Fergusson gives her feedback: "Rachel's diet is varied and of good quality, which is important. So she should try to eat every three to four hours to get glucose to her brain, to fuel it and keep her mind focused and sharp.

"However, Rachel's meals are centred on animal rather than vegetable-based protein, which will make her digestive system sluggish. Vegetarian options such as avocado and chickpeas are anti-inflammatory and easier to digest. She should aim for only 20% of her diet to be from animal proteins.

"The beetroot smoothie was the best breakfast option of the week. The body detoxes and cleanses at night, so giving it something acidic like the grains and dairy in the muesli can upset it. Opt for a vegetable smoothie; your body can absorb more nutrients first thing and it will prevent a sugar or caffeine spike from breakfasts like cereals and coffee. Otherwise, *c'est bon!*"

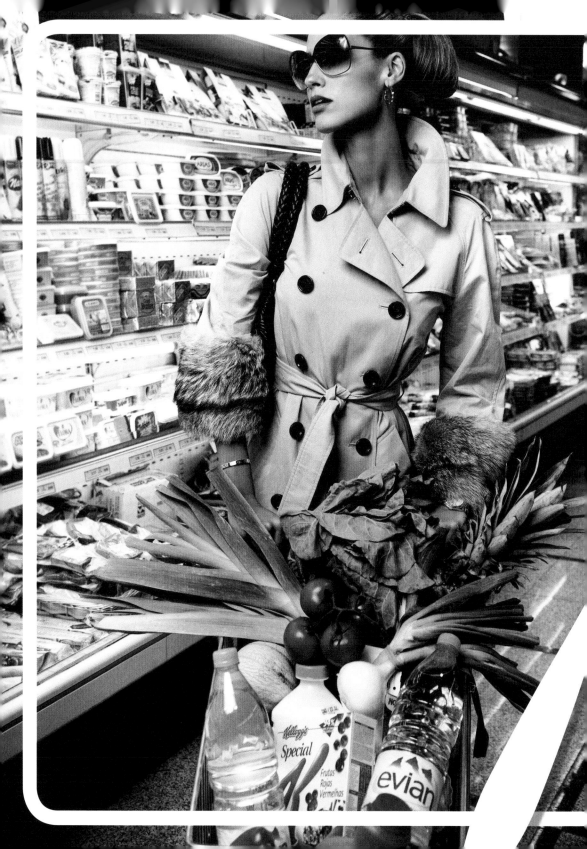

CHAPTER 2

SHOP SMARTER

We enjoy more grocery options these days than ever before, but when you're trying to eat healthily, freedom of choice can lead to information overload. Wholegrain or wholemeal? Low or reduced fat? You can end up unwittingly reversing your good work. Thankfully, our experts have the intel to help you enjoy food, guilt-free – and lose weight with every decision you make.

Your slim-down supermarket secrets

Shopping for flat belly foods can mean a minefield of options. But load up your basket with confidence – we've taken the guesswork out of groceries to help you make the best choices

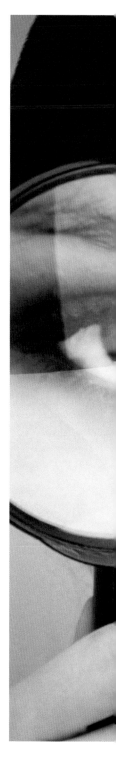

You make a head-spinning 200-plus decisions about food every day, say researchers at Cornell University. And we don't have to tell you that each of these decisions is a new opportunity to do right by your body. To help you eat your way to weight loss we've got the solutions to some everyday food conundrums.

Q WHAT ABOUT BREAKFAST: BROWN TOAST OR MUESLI?

A Munch on muesli, says dietitian Kristen Beck. Every spoonful fuels your body with complex carbs, vitamins, minerals, fibre and calcium from the milk. Just avoid brands that list sugar in the first three ingredients, and keep toasted and cluster varieties to a minimum, as these pack more calories. Check the label to make sure fat content is no more than 5 to 7 per cent; and salt shouldn't exceed 1g per 100g. Three other good low-fat, low-salt cereals to try: Shredded Wheat, Kellogg's Raisin Wheats or Asda Vitality.

Q WHAT'S THE BEST SNACKING STRATEGY FOR ME?

A Every time you eat, invoke the power of three. Each snack should contain protein, fibre and vitamins. So have your cheese with cherry tomatoes and grapes; houmous with carrots and some wholemeal crackers; or a hard-boiled egg with a banana and nuts. Hell, eat the odd Mars Bar – just have it with milk and an apple. This approach works because it makes you conscious of your decisions, helping you avoid snacking mindlessly, says dietitian Karen Beerbower. You may end up eating a few more calories, but you'll feel fuller for longer – and maybe get some extra antioxidants into your system while you're at it.

Q WHAT'S THE BEST OPTION: TOMATO SAUCE OR MUSTARD?

A Smear Colman's on your sausages: "Mustard has more protein, fibre,

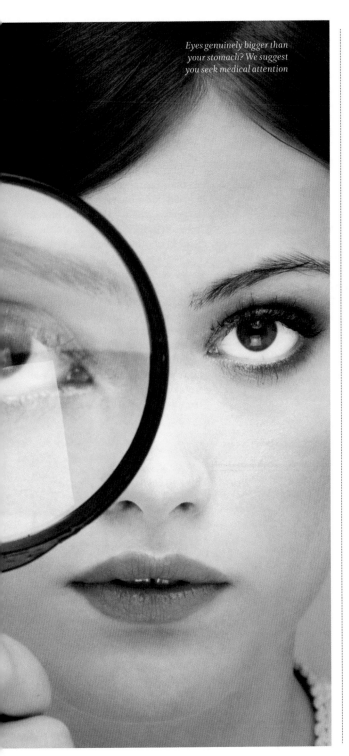

Eyes genuinely bigger than your stomach? We suggest you seek medical attention

calcium, magnesium, potassium, zinc, iron, copper, manganese, selenium and B vitamins, plus less sugar than tomato sauce," says Dr Luise Light, author of *What to Eat.* Not a sausage fan? Add a teaspoon of mustard seeds to your next curry.

Q DOES THE CUT OF MEAT MAKE THAT MUCH DIFFERENCE?

A Yes. Choosing cuts from the leg or loin of an animal will shave fat and calories off your meat and two veg. The least healthy cut is the fatty rib-eye. To tell your shin from shank, download the Ask The Butcher app (£1.49).

Every time you eat, invoke the power of three

Q IS IT TRUE THAT MICROWAVING DESTROYS NUTRIENTS?

A No. In fact, a study in the journal *Nutrition and Food Science* found that microwaving vegetables helps them retain up to 20 per cent more vitamins than hob-cooking them. But it has a dark side. Some plastic containers can leach toxic, potentially carcinogenic chemicals into your meal if you skip the crockery and microwave food in them. "If you wouldn't heat the container and contents in a conventional oven, don't put it in the microwave," says food scientist Dr Daryl Lund.

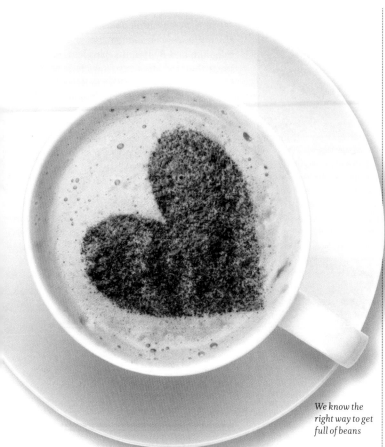

We know the right way to get full of beans

Q DOES IT MATTER WHICH FOODS I EAT FOR PROTEIN?

Yes. Unlike most plant sources of protein, animal protein is "complete", says Dr Donald Layman, professor of nutrition at Illinois State University, US. This means it contains the essential amino acids your body can't synthesise on its own. For a powerful protein punch, try cod – it has around 20g of protein per 100g and just 0.5g of fat. Serve with broccoli to get even more benefits. The Institute of Food Research in Norwich found that eating selenium-rich foods, like cod, with sulforaphane (found in broccoli) increases their cancer-fighting properties by 13 times. If you're a vegan, up your nut roast intake to get your muscles the support they need. You need to

ADDITIONAL RESEARCH: ALICE TRELOAR. ILLUSTRATIONS: LISA BARLOW.

Q WHAT'S MY WAKER-UPPER: COFFEE OR AN ENERGY DRINK?

Coffee, every time. The jolt you feel from an energy drink comes mostly from sugar, which, aside from adding calories, sets you up for an inevitable crash. According to research, frequent coffee breaks (cups of 250ml or less) are the key to sustained alertness rather than one Starbucks Venti Cappuccino (around 600ml), so start with a small coffee and keep it flowing until early afternoon.

> Stick with coffee: the jolt you feel from an energy drink will be mostly from sugar

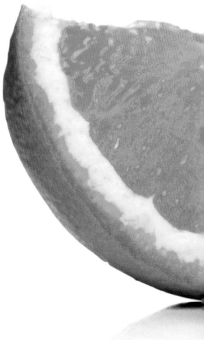

consume 20 to 25 per cent more plant-based protein to reap the same benefits that animal protein sources provide, says nutritionist Dr Mark Tarnopolsky. Nutty, but true.

Q WHAT SHOULD I LOOK FOR WHEN BUYING YOGHURT?

A Go natural, and don't think that fat-free is always the best option. "Almost without exception, 'diet' yoghurts are artificially sweetened and contain additives to simulate the creamy consistency of regular yoghurts," says dietitian Dr Joanna McMillan. Check the nutrition panel and choose one that contains less than 100 calories, 4g of fat and 12g of sugars per 100g. And make sure it has live cultures. "Probiotic bacteria play an essential role in the function of the gut," says Dr McMillan.

Don't miss out on fibre – an essential ingredient for your weight loss goals

Q IS A GLASS OF JUICE AS GOOD AS EATING THE FRUIT WHOLE?

A Not even close. Most prepared fruit juices contain not only natural sugar but lots of added sugar, too. You'll also miss out on fibre – an essential ingredient for your weight loss goals. For example, a medium orange has 62 calories, 12g of sugar, and 3g of belly-filling fibre compared to the 110 calories, 24g of sugar, and zero fibre found in your average glass of OJ. To make juices less sugar-riffic, pour half a glass, then fill the rest with still or carbonated water. You'll be hydrated and healthy.

Q IS CHICKEN A BETTER PROTEIN SOURCE THAN BEEF?

A Not always. A lot depends on how the animals were raised. Today, the average piece of chicken has 266 per cent more fat than it did in 1971, while its protein content has dropped by a third, says research from London

Metropolitan University. So if you can, choose organic-fed, pasture-raised chicken. Similarly, grass-fed beef has 27 per cent less fat than the conventional corn-fed kind. Look for a layer of firm, creamy-white fat on the outside of a steak as a sign of a well-reared animal.

Q SHOULD I DITCH EGG YOLKS IF I WANT TO LOSE WEIGHT?

A No. Super-skinny A-listers may brunch on egg white omelettes, but they're missing out on the best part. Eat the yolks to benefit from vitamin D, choline, carotenoids and the amino acids tryptophan

Today, the average piece of chicken has 266% more fat than it did in 1971

and tyrosine, which have high antioxidant properties to support your body's fat burning ability. Yes, yolks are high in cholesterol, but not the kind that clogs your arteries. Add chopped pepper and parsley when you scramble eggs to up the fibre content and make breakfast even healthier.

Q IS BROWN RICE REALLY THAT MUCH HEALTHIER THAN WHITE?

A Yes, and that goes for all grains. Wholewheat pasta, bread and rice are full of fibre because they're made from the entire kernel. If the fibre is taken out – as is the case with white rice and bread – fast-rising blood sugar triggers your pancreas to release insulin, the hormone that lowers blood sugar and signals your body to store fat. In fact, replace just one 50g serving of white rice with brown a week, and you'll cut your risk of type 2 diabetes by 16 per cent, say researchers from the Harvard School of Public Health.

Q WHAT'S THE BEST OPTION: A HOTDOG OR A SLICE OF PIZZA?

A Basically, the more high-fibre vegetables you can include, the better, so a pizza is probably your

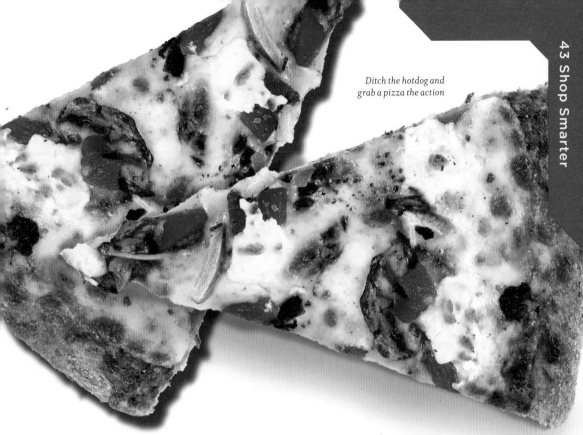

Ditch the hotdog and grab a pizza the action

best option. It's not a perfect meal – the carbs in the base will probably be the unhealthy refined type, but if you order a pizza topped with spinach, mushrooms, peppers or rocket you'll be getting some valuable nutrients. Not to mention a hefty shot of cancer-fighting lycopene from the cooked tomatoes. Try Pizza Express' Leggera range; they have half the base of normal pizzas which means only 500 calories and less than 5g of saturated fat.

Some fruit loses as much as 25% of its vitamin C after six days in the fridge

Q FOR HOW LONG DOES FRESH FRUIT STAY NUTRITIOUS?

A For as long as it looks appetising. "In general, fresh-cut fruits tend to visually spoil before significant nutrient loss occurs," says food scientist Dr Maria Gil. So if it looks a bit off, the chances are its vitamins might well will be, too. Her research in the *Journal of Agriculture and Food Chemistry* found that some fruits lose as much as 25 per cent of their vitamin C and carotenoids after six days of refrigeration, with cantaloupe and pineapple the fastest to deteriorate. So be selective about what you buy and when; don't buy fruit in bulk and make sure you eat fruit within a week of it ripening **WH**

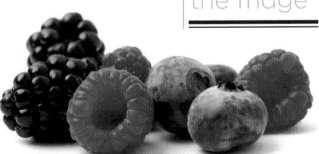

Outfox the box

Food companies use every trick in the book to make you eat more. Improve your label literacy and you'll find you lose weight without even trying.

Here's the speediest weight-loss tip we've ever heard: pick up a product, turn it over and scan the small print on the back. "Reading labels is one of the top five things you can do to improve the way you eat," says British Dietetic Association dietitian Sian Porter. Deceptive packaging claims and "creative" serving sizes mean you're eating more than you realise – and that starts from the first meal of the day. So we asked nutrition experts for some fail-safe decoding strategies. Read 'em and reap the slimline rewards.

1 AVOID THE NATURAL TRAP

Research shows we eat more of foods with packaging peppered with meaningless phrases like "All natural". Don't be sucked in. For example, "A good source of" means the product contains 10-20% of your daily requirement for the mentioned nutrient. In other words, you'd need 5 to 10 servings to get your full day's value.

2 TRUST SPECIFIC CLAIMS

"Any food that wants to carry a health claim – for example, that it lowers cholesterol levels – now has to meet stringent European Commission guidelines, so you can have confidence in them," says dietitian Helen Bond of the British Dietetic Association. But be careful with wishy-washy words. 'Multigrain', for example, just means that more than one type of grain is used – they may still be heavily refined. A more trustworthy grain claim is "100 per cent wholemeal".

3 DON'T BE TOO COLOUR BLIND

The traffic light symbols make things super-easy: green is good; red is bad. However, don't follow this at the expense of variety in your diet – some foods like cheese will never have a "green" rating for fat so just be sensible with portion sizes (think matchbox, not pack of cards).

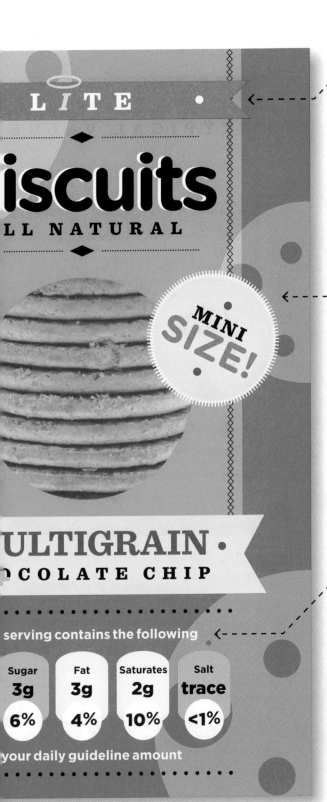

LITE

iscuits

LL NATURAL

MINI SIZE!

ULTIGRAIN •

COLATE CHIP

serving contains the following

Sugar	Fat	Saturates	Salt
3g	**3g**	**2g**	**trace**
6%	4%	10%	<1%

your daily guideline amount

4 MOVE AWAY FROM THE 'LITE'

"Research shows that people over-consume diet products," says Porter. "When you see 'reduced-fat', 'lite' or 'light' on a label it just means it's 30% less than the standard product, not that it's fat free. In a high-fat product like mayonnaise, there will still be a lot of fat." Here's a much better idea: compare the calorie count per 100g to a non-diet version – there's often little difference.

5 DON'T MAX OUT ON MINIS

"It's easy to overeat miniature items. Our minds equate the small size with fewer calories," says Young. Take Mini Cheddars – if you eat the whole 50g bag, you'll take in 258 calories and 15g fat, whereas four full-sized Cheddars only have 80 calories and 4.8g fat. And you'll benefit from choosing full-size products in big bags. Dutch research found people ate twice as many crisps if they came in small, rather than large, packets.

6 CHECK THE SERVING SIZE

"We don't have a standard portion size in the UK, so look at what you're eating – does it serve one or two?" says Porter. If the ready meal gives values per half pack, immediately put the other half in a container in the fridge, then fill up the rest of your plate with salad or veg.

❯

MIND THE BACK

Welcome to the flip side. Here's how to make sense of nutrition labels to shed weight, not brain cells.

TYPICAL VALUE

	100g contains	Each biscuit contains	%GDA*	GDA* for a ty... adult
Energy	2080kJ 500kcal	240kJ 60kcal	3%	2000k...
Protein	5.1g	0.6g		
Carbohydrates	67.9g	7.9g		
of which sugars	28.4g	3g	6%	50g
Fat	23g	3g	4%	70g
of which saturates	13.7g	2g	10%	20g
mono-unsaturates	6.7g	0.8g		
polyunsaturates	2g	0.2g		
Fibre	2.1g	0.2g		
Sodium	0.2g	trace		
Salt equivalent	0.5g	trace	<1%	6g

*Guideline daily amounts

1 GO THE PRO
"As a rule, 20 per cent of your energy should come from protein," says dietitian Molly Morgan. That's around 400 calories a day from protein. The best choices: skinless white meat, seafood and low-fat dairy.

2 FACE FAT FACTS
To be legally classed as low-fat, a product must have 3g fat or less per 100g, says Bond. But it's the type of fat that's more important – steer clear of trans-fatty acids (aka "hydrogenated vegetable fats"), and look for foods with no more than 1.5g saturated fat per 100g.

3 EASE OFF ON SALT
Around 75% of salt in our diets comes from processed foods, so avoid anything with more than 1.5g per 100g. Sandwiches or ready meals should have 1.25g or less. If a product only gives the sodium values, then multiply them by 2.5 to get the salt content.

Wheat flour, sugar, vegetable oil, whey solids, glucose syrup, wheat starch, salt, raising agents (ammonium bicarbonate, sodium bicarbonate), corn starch, vanillin, natural flavouring

**CONTAINS: WHEAT, MILK, GLUTEN
MAY ALSO CONTAIN TRACES OF NUTS**

500g

4 GO COMPLEX

With carbohydrate-rich products (bread, pasta, rice) look for products that contain low-GI complex carbs says nutritionist Kristen Beck. How to tell if they're complex: "They'll have a high carb value but low sugar value in the nutrition panel."

5 DO THE MATHS

Sugar is converted into fat by your liver. So you need to know how much you're ingesting. To do this, divide the number in grams by 4 to give you the equivalent in teaspoons. That means a 500ml bottle of innocuous sounding Glaceau Vitamin Multi-V Water (23g sugar) packs nearly six teaspoons. Ouch.

6 SUSS OUT SUGAR

Sugar hides in labels under many names. The most common is words ending in "ose" (like fructose) but also watch out for: cane juice, corn syrup, diastatic malt, diatase, disaccharide, erythritol, fruit juice concentrate, fruit syrup, glycerol, molasses, monsaccharide, rice extract and sorbitol.

7 ORDER, ORDER

By law, labels have to list ingredients in order of volume. So if the first ingredient is sugar that's probably pretty bad. (Unless, of course, it's a bag of sugar). And do a count – foods with five ingredients or fewer are your best option WH

* THE GUIDELINE DAILY AMOUNT FOR WOMEN IS 2000 CALORIES A DAY, ACCORDING TO THE BRITISH DIETETIC ASSOCIATION.

KNOW YOUR LIMITS

Easy guidelines for the average UK woman* to stick to:

Our experts have created this diagram to help you decipher how many calories to eat at each meal. We've even allowed a couple of snacks...

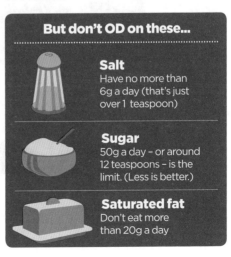

Snacks
2 x 200 calories

Breakfast
400 calories

TOTAL
2000 calories

Dinner
600 calories

Lunch
600 calories

But don't OD on these...

Salt
Have no more than 6g a day (that's just over 1 teaspoon)

Sugar
50g a day – or around 12 teaspoons – is the limit. (Less is better.)

Saturated fat
Don't eat more than 20g a day

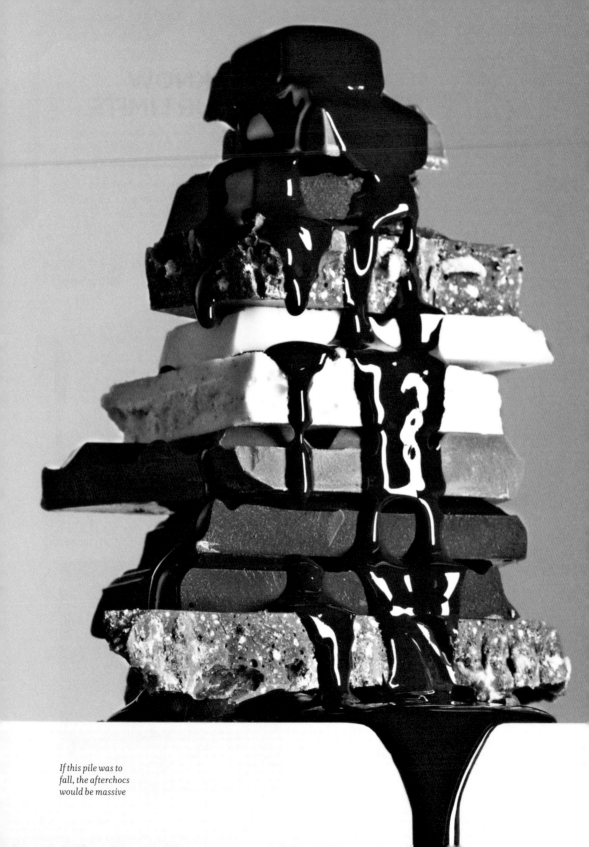

If this pile was to fall, the afterchocs would be massive

Choc value

When the craving strikes, it's easy to be blinded by the 'healthy' options on the chocolate shelf. But which really hit the nutritional sweet spot?

RAW

The Katherine Jenkins of chocolate, raw seems so perfect, we're a little suspicious. The science goes thus; because the ingredients are treated below 46°C, its antioxidant content is retained.

I SHOULD COCOA Our nutritionist Christy Fergusson says: "The US Department of Agriculture tested the antioxidant content of different chocolates and raw was rated 1,200% more potent than dark – and 6,000% better than the milk kind." Plus, raw bars don't have refined sugar and their fat content primarily comes from natural fats.

THE DARK SIDE While raw uses its powers for good (34% of its fat is monounsaturated oleic acid, shown to decrease the risk of heart disease), its fat content is often higher than that of milk choc. So if you're thinking, "It's a superfood, what's the problem?" – er, that's it.

ORGANIC

If your bar is labelled organic, it simply means that 95% of its grown ingredients meet the organic standard of a regulatory body – in the UK's case that's often the Soil Association.

I SHOULD COCOA "Organic is 'good' in terms of what it doesn't give you – namely cacao beans grown using pesticides or cow's milk affected by antibiotics," says Fergusson. And since ingredients may be higher quality (one US study showed organic milk had 62% more omega-3 fatty acids than standard milk), you'll likely be getting a better standard of bar.

THE DARK SIDE Studies show that when people see an organic label on food, they often assume it's lower in calories. "Sadly, organic bars are just as calorific as Dairy Milk, and packed with similar sugar and fat content," Fergusson warns. At least the cows are happy.

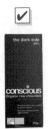

EAT THIS

Conscious The Dark Side 85%, 50g (£2.50, 310 cals, 85% cacao)

A hit of antioxidants and dietary fibre to slow absorption of its agave. Perfection.

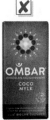

NOT THAT

Ombar Coco Mylk, 35g (£1.99, 190 cals 60% cacao)

Failing on a technicality, this bar's 60% cacao means we downgraded it to second place.

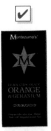

EAT THIS

Montezuma's Orange & Geranium, 100g (£2.39, 548 cals, 73% cacao)

Yes, this bar is organic, but it also goes above and beyond with its 73% cacoa content. Winner.

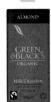

NOT THAT

Green and Black's Organic Almond, 100g (£2.00, 578 cals, 37% cacao)

Protein-rich almonds are a plus, but with 38% sugar and 37% cacao it's just not good enough.

If this doesn't make you join the dark side, we don't know what will

DARK

Here's a shocker: EU legislation means UK chocolate must only contain 35% cocoa solids to be termed dark. In reality, no bar dares claim that mantle unless it's 50%.

I SHOULD COCOA "The antioxidants really kick in at 85%," says Fergusson. "But if you can't handle it that dark, 60 to 70% is still better than milk, as its proteins bind to antioxidant flavonoids making them unavailable to the body." Secondly: dark has less sugar. Green and Black's Dark contains 13.5g sugar per 100g, while their milk bar has more than three times that at 45.5g.

THE DARK SIDE Levels of the chemical compound theobromine can be 10 times higher in dark chocolate than milk, which isn't great if you're prone to skin conditions such as acne. Theobromine is thought to have pore-clogging properties. Bummer.

✔	✘
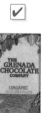	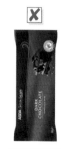
EAT THIS	**NOT THAT**
The Grenada Chocolate Company, 85g (£3.35, 570 cals, 100% cacao)	*Asda Dark Chocolate, 200g (£1.00, 515 cals per 100g, 50% cacao)*
The only way to eat a bar this bitter is to let it melt on your tongue.	Barely scraping into the dark category, this has 47% sugar. Uh oh.

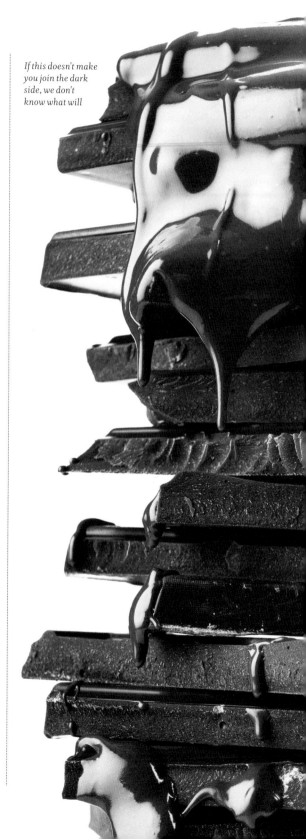

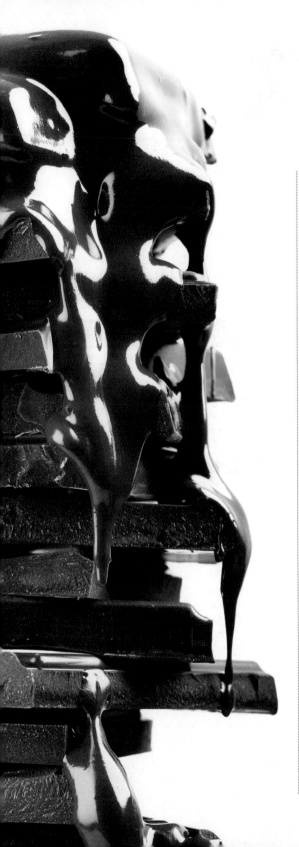

With a GI of zero, stevia won't send you on a sugar spike

NO ADDED SUGAR

Sugar: harder to avoid than your ex on a fat day, so no-added-sugar labels are rare. "Legally, a bar can only be no-added-sugar if it doesn't contain absorbable calories from sugar," says nutritionist Drew Price.

I SHOULD COCOA Stevia is the current go-to natural sugar substitute – and for very good reason. With a GI of zero – yes, zero – it won't send you on a sugar roller coaster. Moreover, a study in the journal *Appetite* found that people said they felt more satisfied by snacks flavoured with stevia than those who ate regular sugary ones. They also recorded lower insulin levels after the stevia treat. Sweet.

THE DARK SIDE "You're more likely to lose out on antioxidants by opting for a no-added-sugar bar," says Price. "Unless you need to cut sugar completely, have a couple of squares of raw chocolate instead – its dietary fibre will slow down sugar absorption." WH

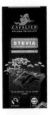

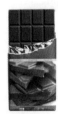

EAT THIS	NOT THAT
Cavalier Rice Crisp Dark, 40g (£1.69, 431 cals per 100g, 55% cacao)	*Boots No Added Sugar Swiss Chocolate, 100g (£1.99, 554 cals, 53% cacao)*
With flaxseed and stevia, this has got super elements sewn in.	Contains aspartame, which can rob your body of vital nutrients.

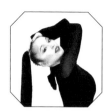

MY FLAT BELLY DIARY:

Nicole Winhoffer

Celebrity trainer Nicole Winhoffer is the woman behind Madonna's age-defying body. How does she cram healthy eating into her busy schedule?

MONDAY

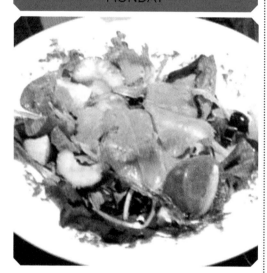

8am
All-Bran with soy milk, an espresso and water

12pm
Smoked salmon with green salad, olives, avocado, cucumbers and tomatoes

7pm
Pumpkin soup

7:30pm
Grilled chicken with steamed vegetables

I take a lot of supplements. One of my favourites is apple pectin, which is apparently good for burning fat. My doctor also advised me to take omega-3 and iron, which will support my body through all the exercise I do – it can range between 12 and 14 hours a week.

TUESDAY

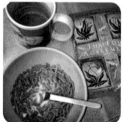

7:45am
All-Bran and a coffee, both with soy milk

11am
Peanut butter protein bar

3pm
Brown rice cake

7pm
Wholewheat turkey sandwich with mustard

9pm
Organic roasted almonds

I travelled a lot this week, including a 30-hour flight. I grabbed food en route and on the plane, but I prefer to eat proper meals because when I start snacking, I just want to eat all day long.

WEDNESDAY

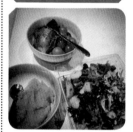

8am
Spelt flakes and a coffee, both with almond milk

11am
Peanut butter protein bar

3pm
Greek yoghurt

5pm
Tuna Niçoise salad with tomatoes, puréed carrots, parsnips, steamed spinach and half an avocado

I eat some carbs and protein at least an hour and a half before training and then afterwards. Protein helps to rebuild muscle. I'm usually quite strict with my diet on weekdays.

AS TOLD TO: AMELIA JEAN JONES. PHOTOGRAPHY: ADAM RINDY/HCF. ORGANIC FOOD BARS, £24 FOR 12, EVOLUTIONORGANICS.CO.UK

THURSDAY	FRIDAY	SATURDAY	SUNDAY

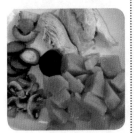 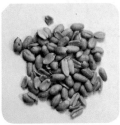 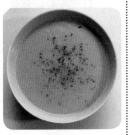 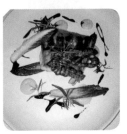

THURSDAY	FRIDAY	SATURDAY	SUNDAY
8am *All-Bran and a coffee, both with almond milk* **12pm** *Peanut butter protein bar* **2pm** *Greek yoghurt* **5pm** *Steamed chicken, mushrooms and butternut squash with avocado and beetroot*	**9am** *Spelt flakes with almond milk* **2pm** *Brown rice cakes* **5pm** *Skinless roast chicken with steamed vegetables and tomatoes* **6:30pm** *A handful of unsalted peanuts with green tea*	**7:30am** *All-Bran cereal without milk and a black coffee* **11am** *2 litres water* **12:30pm** *2 tbsp all-natural peanut butter* **2pm** *Grilled chicken breast with brown rice and oiled veg* **6pm** *Pumpkin soup*	**9am** *All-Bran cereal and a coffee* **10am** *Roasted nuts* **1:15pm** *Grilled chicken with spinach salad, avocado, broccoli and lemon dressing* **3pm** *Greek yoghurt* **6pm** *Grilled fish with chicory*
I do two sessions a week with my PT. A mid-afternoon snack gives me the boost I need. I do 30 minutes on the treadmill and bike, then I work on core exercises.	I change my diet every six months, according to research I've done online. I like to test things out on myself and record changes in my body and energy levels.	I did an hour of toning and 45 minutes of cardio today. I target one area of my body per week with 15 full-body exercises using weights, bands or dumbbells.	Breakfast is glucose-based, low in fat and high in fibre and protein. I have an active day so I need the morning carbs for the energy, I'll burn throughout the day.

THE EXPERT VERDICT

Our nutritionist Dr Christy Fergusson gives her opinion: "Although Nicole is mindful of what she eats, she does often skip lunch and dinner and opt for protein bars and snacks instead.

"Switching her cereal to an alkalising, low-glycaemic green juice and eating lunch would make her less likely to snack.

"Meanwhile, replacing coffee with yerba mate tea would give her an energy boost without being overstimulating.

"Nicole should also consider swapping peanut butter for almond butter if she craves something sweet, as it's lower in saturated fat but is still packed with a nutty flavour. And while

cooking without oil or butter cuts fat, she could use coconut oil, which is thermogenic, making it great for weight loss.

"She should try organic protein bars that are made from organic ingredients. They're raw, nutrient-dense and are a good protein source – great for someone as busy as Nicole."

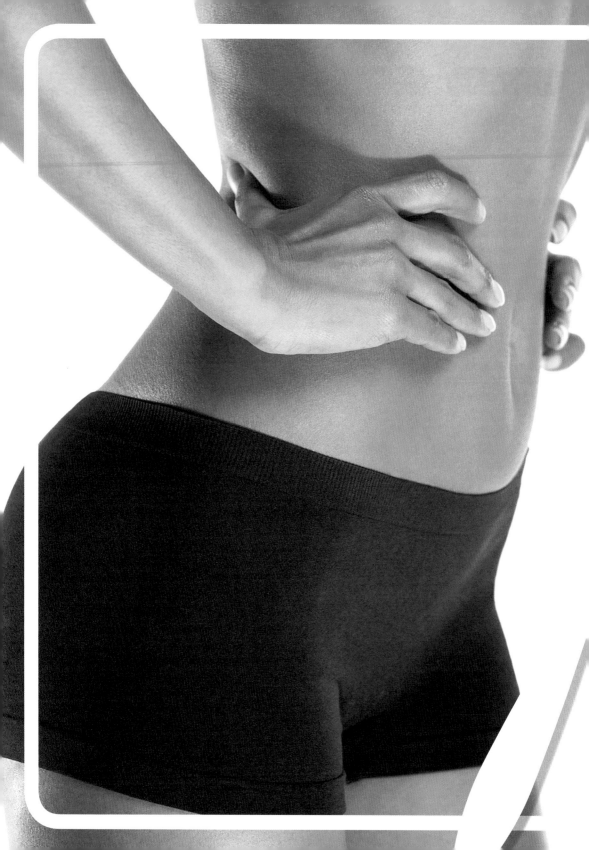

YOUR FLAT BELLY FORTNIGHT

Despite being big fans of long-term healthy eating, we know there are times when you need to fast-track your weight loss. This healthy, delicious eating plan is designed to help you lose two pounds in just 14 days, with a varied menu that will keep you full at all times but adds up to just 1500 calories a day. Magic.

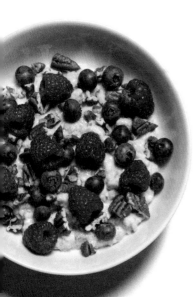

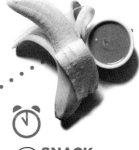

1 BREAKFAST
PORRIDGE WITH PECANS AND BERRIES

- 1 packet Original Quaker Instant Oat So Simple
- 180ml skimmed milk
- 30g chopped pecans
- 100g raspberries
- 100g blueberries

BELLY BENEFIT
The raspberries bag 6.5g of fibre – that's a quarter of your RDA. Plus, soluble fibre in porridge will keep you feeling full past lunch
TOTAL 351 CALORIES

2 SNACK
PEANUT BUTTER WITH BANANA

- 1 medium banana
- 2 tsp peanut butter

BELLY BENEFIT
Studies have found eating protein-rich nuts in the morning leads to consuming fewer calories during the day.
TOTAL 167 CALORIES

Week 1: Monday

Start as you mean to go on with filling, lean protein and antioxidant-packed berries to give your system a boost. And yes, you're even allowed chocolate

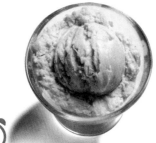

6 EXTRA SNACK
GYM REWARD ICE CREAM

- 2 scoops (125ml) Kelly's Clotted Cream Cornish Ice Cream

HAVE THIS IF...
You've exercised for at least 30 minutes today.
TOTAL 135 CALORIES

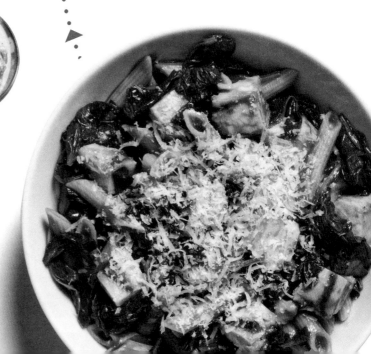

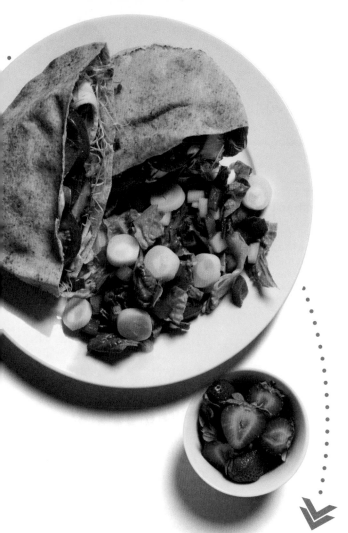

3 LUNCH
TURKEY PITTA WITH SALAD AND STRAWBERRIES

- 110g fresh roast turkey
- 1 tsp Dijon mustard
- 50g baby spinach leaves
- 1 small tomato, sliced
- 1 small handful alfalfa sprouts
- 1 small wholewheat pitta
- 1 cup chopped romaine lettuce
- ½ small cucumber, sliced
- 1 red pepper, chopped
- ½ tin Green Giant hearts of palm, chopped
- 1 tsp olive oil
- 60g strawberries

BELLY BENEFIT
Of all animal proteins, turkey has the least calories per 30g. Like dairy, it also contains the amino acid leucine which is thought to play a role in preserving muscle mass during weight loss. So you'll lose weight while keeping your metabolism running at full speed.

TOTAL 395 CALORIES

4 SNACK
CHOCOLATE CINNALATTE

- Skinny latte sprinkled with cinnamon powder
- 2 pieces Lindt Excellence 70% chocolate

BELLY BENEFIT
The flavonols in dark chocolate boost HDL (ie, good) cholesterol levels. Plus, cinnamon helps control insulin, keeping your blood sugar steady.
TOTAL 150 CALORIES

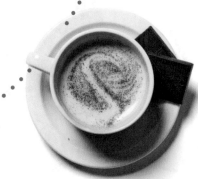

5 DINNER
CHICKEN AND SPINACH PENNE

- 110g grilled chicken, chopped into small pieces
- 125ml tomato sauce
- 250g baby spinach leaves
- 115g wholewheat penne
- 1½ tbsp grated Parmesan

BELLY BENEFIT
Fibre is the key to losing weight without hunger – and spinach is a low-cal way to up your intake. To preserve nutrients, stir the spinach leaves into the pasta sauce one minute before serving.
TOTAL 437 CALORIES

PHOTOGRAPHY: JEFF HARRIS.

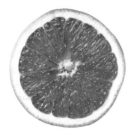

1 BREAKFAST
AVOCADO AND EGG ON TOAST WITH GRAPEFRUIT

- 2 medium grapefruit
- 1 slice wholegrain toast
- 1 egg, fried or poached
- ½ avocado, sliced

BELLY BENEFIT
Start the day with a citrus twist. A study found eating grapefruit before each meal helped adults lose almost half a kilogram in 12 weeks, without making any other dietary changes.
TOTAL 380 CALORIES

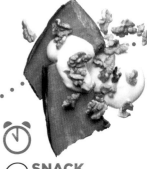

2 SNACK
SWEET POTATO

- ½ medium jacket sweet potato
- 60g plain low-fat yoghurt
- 1½ tbsp chopped walnuts

BELLY BENEFIT
Studies have shown that eating low-GI foods, such as sweet potato, helps reduce body fat.
TOTAL 157 CALORIES

Week 1: Tuesday

Don't let your tastebuds won't get bored. Get zesty with grapefruit, feel the burn with sweet potato and get to the gym to score a glass of wine

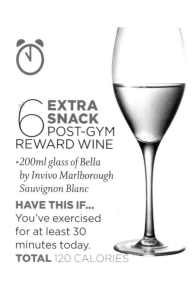

6 EXTRA SNACK
POST-GYM REWARD WINE

- 200ml glass of Bella by Invivo Marlborough Sauvignon Blanc

HAVE THIS IF...
You've exercised for at least 30 minutes today.
TOTAL 120 CALORIES

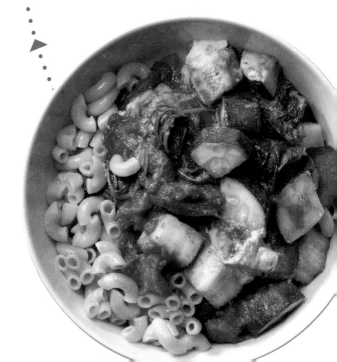

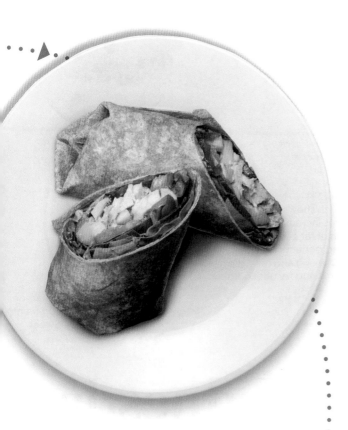

3 LUNCH CHICKEN SALAD WRAP

- 1 wholemeal wrap
- 85g chicken breast
- 1 celery stalk, chopped
- 1 apple, chopped
- 2 tsp olive oil
- 1 tsp Dijon mustard
- Baby spinach leaves
- 2 slices tomato

BELLY BENEFIT
Chicken is a top source of tryptophan which helps to lower levels of cortisol, the crafty culprit for tubby 'stress' bellies. Add lots of salad vegetables, too; the fibre content fills you up with a minimal calorie intake.
TOTAL 379 CALORIES

5 DINNER CHEESY VEGGIE PASTA

- 60g wholewheat macaroni
- 1 tin low-salt tomatoes
- 140g low-fat ricotta cheese
- 40g spinach, chopped
- 1 courgette, chopped
- 2 tsp olive oil

BELLY BENEFIT
Low-fat dairy, such as ricotta, helps to keep your weight in check – as does having a meat-free day at least once a week, according to a recent study in *The American Journal of Clinical Nutrition*.
TOTAL 439 CALORIES

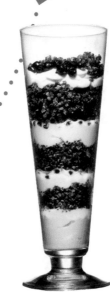

4 SNACK CURRANT SUNDAE

- 100g plain low-fat yoghurt
- 70g cooked quinoa
- 2 tsp blackcurrants

BELLY BENEFIT
100g yoghurt has just as much hunger-quashing protein as an egg. Meanwhile, nutrient-rich quinoa packs amino acid lysine, which is essential for muscle repair – and perfect for gym bunnies.
TOTAL 145 CALORIES

PHOTOGRAPHY: LEVI BROWN.

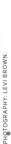
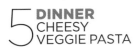

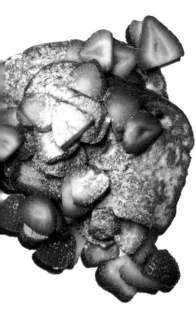

1 BREAKFAST
FRENCH TOAST WITH SUGARED STRAWBERRIES

- 1 egg
- 1 tbsp skimmed milk
- 2 slices wholemeal bread
- 13 strawberries, sliced
- ½ tsp icing sugar

BELLY BENEFIT
New research shows eating strawberries increases your production of fat-burning hormone adiponectin. For the toast, mix the egg and milk, dip the bread in it and fry until golden.
TOTAL 275 CALORIES

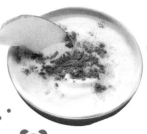

2 SNACK
APPLE WITH YOGHURT

- 1 apple, sliced
- 125g low-fat plain yoghurt
- ¼ tsp cinnamon powder

BELLY BENEFIT
The polyphenols in cinnamon help regulate blood sugar and keep hunger at bay. Sweet.
TOTAL 155 CALORIES

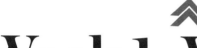

Week 1: Wednesday

Fry away any unwanted stomach fat by following this easy-to-prepare, oh-so satisfying meal plan

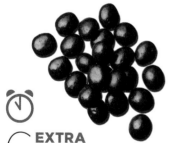

6 EXTRA SNACK
CHOCOLATE ESPRESSO BEANS

- 28g choc-covered (dark) espresso beans

HAVE THIS IF...
You've exercised for at least 30 minutes today.
TOTAL 120 CALORIES

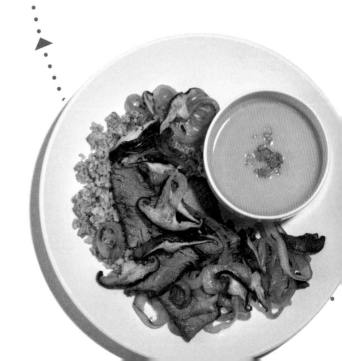

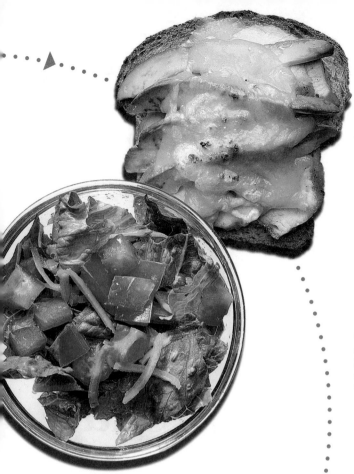

3 LUNCH
GRILLED CHICKEN AND AVOCADO MELT

- 1 slice wholemeal bread
- 85g grilled chicken breast
- ¼ avocado, thinly sliced
- 28g low-fat cheddar
- ½ onion, sliced

SIDE SALAD
- 100g tomatoes, lettuce, carrots and a drizzle of olive oil

BELLY BENEFIT
In an Australian study, dieters who ate five helpings a day of cheese and other dairy foods lost more belly fat than those who ate three. Grate result.
TOTAL 438 CALORIES

5 DINNER
SQUASH SOUP AND STIR-FRY

- 150g Glorious! New England Butternut Squash Skinny Soup
- 85g tenderloin fillet steak, sliced
- 160g cooked bulgar
- 120g shiitake mushrooms, sliced
- ½ onion, sliced
- 2 tsp olive oil

BELLY BENEFIT
Bulgar, a quick-to-cook, nutty flavoured whole grain, is a great alternative to rice, with about 25 per cent fewer calories.
TOTAL 450 CALORIES

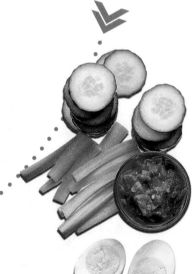

4 SNACK
SALSA CRUDITES

- 100g cucumber, sliced
- 200g carrots, sliced
- 50g salsa for dipping
- 1 large egg, hard-boiled

BELLY BENEFIT
Carrots are packed full of appetite-busting fibre, so crunch on a couple in the afternoon and you'll munch less at dinner.
TOTAL 182 CALORIES

PHOTOGRAPHY: LEVI BROWN

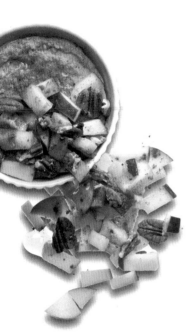

1 BREAKFAST
BAKED OATS WITH APPLE

- 20g steel-cut oats
- 1 tsp baking powder
- 60ml skimmed milk
- 1 egg white
- 3 tbsps apple sauce
- ½ tsp cinnamon
- 2 tsps chopped pecans
- 125g apple, chopped
- 1 tsp honey

Mix the top six ingredients, bake for 6 mins at 180°C. Add other ingredients.

BELLY BENEFIT
Steel-cut oats last longer in the stomach, so you stay full.
TOTAL 320 CALORIES

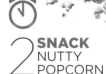

2 SNACK
NUTTY POPCORN

- 10 dry-roasted nuts
- 2 tbsps Parmesan
- 8g air-popped popcorn

BELLY BENEFIT
Studies show nuts help boost production of serotonin – a hormone that reduces appetite and boosts mood.
TOTAL 210 CALORIES

Week 1: Thursday

Today you fuel up with oats, chicken and scallops, and keep your metabolism running with apple, spinach and beetroot. Your body says thanks, by the way

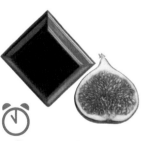

6 EXTRA SNACK
FIGS AND CHOCOLATE

ADD *10g dark chocolate and 1 fig.*
SUBTRACT *The pecans and 1 tbsp Parmesan from the popcorn snack.*
TOTAL 160 CALORIES

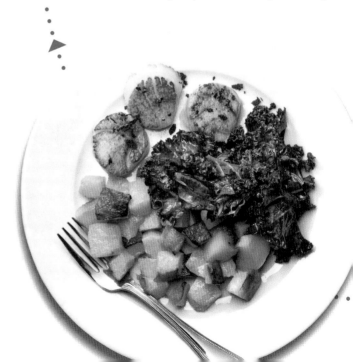

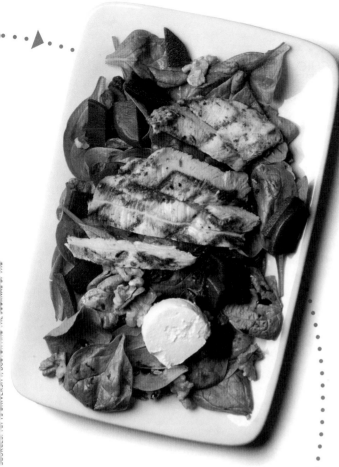

3 LUNCH
CHICKEN, GOAT'S CHEESE AND BEETROOT SALAD

- *260g baby spinach*
- *140g chopped beetroot*
- *1 tbsp dried cranberries*
- *15g walnuts*
- *85g grilled chicken breast*
- *30g goat's cheese*
- *1 tbsp balsamic vinegar*

BELLY BENEFIT
A study in the Journal of Functional Foods found vinegar's acetic acid helps suppress your body fat accumulation and aids weight loss. Salt & Vinegar Chipsticks don't count.
TOTAL 420 CALORIES

5 DINNER
SCALLOPS WITH LEMON AND SAGE

- *85g scallops*
- *2 tsps rapeseed oil*
- *2 tsps lemon juice*
- *½ tsp ground sage*
- *240g cubed roasted squash*
- *140g kale sautéed in 2 tsp olive oil*

Cook the scallops in oil for 2 mins on each side. Drizzle with juice and sage, then serve with the squash and kale.

BELLY BENEFIT
Kaempferol, a flavonoid in kale, helps prevent fat building up around your organs. Flat tummies all round.
TOTAL 350 CALORIES

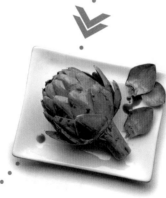

4 SNACK
ARTICHOKE LEAVES IN DRESSING

- *1 cooked artichoke*
- *1 tsp olive oil*
- *50ml balsamic vinegar*

BELLY BENEFIT
A US study found eating a snack in 30 minutes not five increased levels of peptides that leave you fuller for longer. A fiddly artichoke will take time.
TOTAL 200 CALORIES

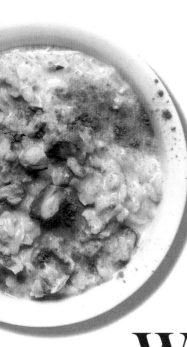

1 BREAKFAST
PISTACHIO RICE PUDDING

· 50g instant brown rice
· 180ml skimmed milk
· 15 pistachios
· 1 tsp brown sugar
· ½ tsp cinnamon

Cook the rice in the milk. Mix in the pistachios, then top with the sugar and cinnamon.

BELLY BENEFIT
A Penn State University study found pistachios help to lower LDL (bad) cholesterol. That's worth shelling out for.
TOTAL 220 CALORIES

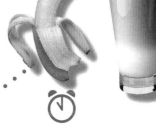

2 SNACK
BANANA AND A LATTE

· 1 large banana
· 350ml skimmed vanilla latte
· ½ tsp cinnamon

BELLY BENEFIT
Caffeine is a double threat to flab. It increases fat burn and revs up your metabolism. Drink up.
TOTAL 280 CALORIES

Week 1: Friday

From this luxurious, slow-burn breakfast to a deceptively low calorie dessert, you're guaranteed that Friday feeling without undoing all your good work

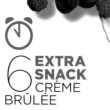

6 EXTRA SNACK
CRÈME BRÛLÉE

ADD Crème brûlée: boil semi-skimmed milk, 3 tbsp Organ Egg Replacer, ½ tsp vanilla, 1 tbsp sugar. Bake at 180°C for 45mins. Top with raspberries.
SUBTRACT Avocado at lunch and half a sausage from dinner.
TOTAL 147 CALORIES

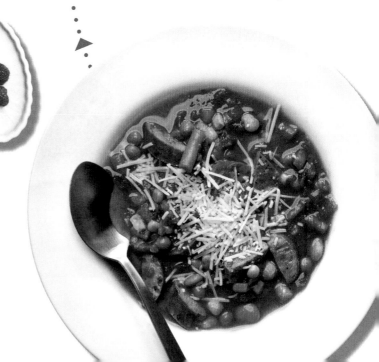

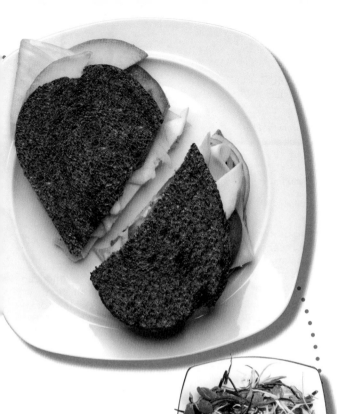

3 LUNCH
TURKEY AND AVOCADO SANDWICH

- 2 slices rye bread
- 1 tbsp French mustard
- 90g skinless turkey breast
- 2 slices tomato
- 1 red onion, sliced
- 40g avocado, sliced

COLESLAW

- 90g red cabbage, shredded
- 2 tbsp raisins
- 1 tbsp low-fat mayonnaise

BELLY BENEFIT
According to *Nutrition Journal*, rye bread has more fibre than whole-wheat bread, so it keeps you full up for longer. Go on, use your loaf.
TOTAL 420 CALORIES

5 DINNER
ITALIAN SAUSAGE AND VEG HOTPOT

- 150g Italian smoked turkey sausage, diced
- 1 tin Baxters Chunky Country Vegetable Soup
- ½ tsp grated Parmesan

BELLY BENEFIT
As well as being a great source of lean protein, turkey also helps to guard against bone fractures. Gobble up!
TOTAL 350 CALORIES

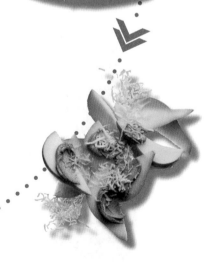

4 SNACK
ALMONDY PEARS WITH COCONUT

- 1 pear, sliced
- 1 tbsp almond butter
- 1½ tbsp shredded coconut

BELLY BENEFIT
Almond cell walls help reduce the amount of fat absorbed by the body. Now that's nuts.
TOTAL 230 CALORIES

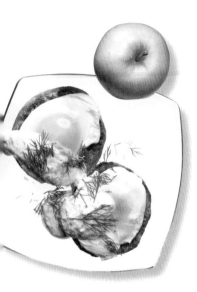

1 BREAKFAST
EGGS BENEDICT AND AN APPLE

- 2 poached eggs
- 3 tbsp 0% fat yoghurt with ¼ tsp dried dill, ¼ tsp lemon juice and ½ tsp lemon zest
- 1 sprig fresh dill
- 1 Kingsmill 50/50 muffin
- 1 small apple

BELLY BENEFIT
Get belly-fighting protein in your diet with eggs. A recent study found people who ate two a day lost 65% more weight than those who had a carby bagel for brekkie.
TOTAL 440 CALORIES

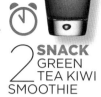

2 SNACK
GREEN TEA KIWI SMOOTHIE

- 2 kiwi fruit
- 1 tbsp honey
- 250ml green tea
- 80ml fat-free vanilla soy milk

BELLY BENEFIT
A study by the American Journal Of Nutrition showed green tea boosts metabolism by 30-40%.
TOTAL 180 CALORIES

Week 1: Saturday

There's no need to let your weight loss goal cramp your style this weekend with a Mexican-inspired lunch and dinner grilled *al fresco*

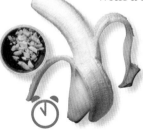

6 EXTRA SNACK
CHOCO-NUT BANANA

ADD *A small banana dipped in chocolate (melt 10g Ombar Organic 72% Bio Live Dark Chocolate) sprinkled with 2 crushed peanuts.*
SUBTRACT *The apple from breakfast and the cheese and yoghurt from lunch. Easy.*
TOTAL 150 CALORIES

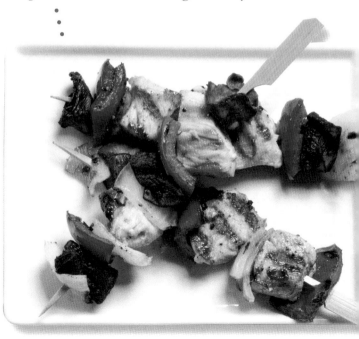

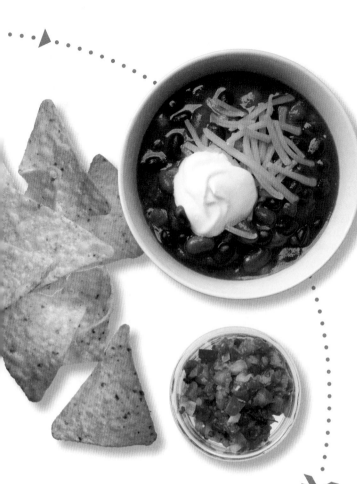

3 LUNCH
BEAN SOUP WITH TORTILLAS AND SALSA

- ½ can Heinz Farmers' Market Three Bean & Pepper Soup
- 2 tbsps non-fat Greek yoghurt
- 2 tbsps grated Cheddar cheese
- 30g low-fat tortilla chips
- 3 tbsps salsa

BELLY BENEFIT
Include yoghurt in your diet for extra flat-belly results. Studies show the calcium helps to maintain muscle mass and increase fat loss. Grab a spoon.
TOTAL 330 CALORIES

4 SNACK
NECTARINE, HONEY AND RICOTTA TOASTS

- 60g low-fat ricotta
- 2 tsps honey
- Ryvita Sweet Onion Crispbread
- 1 small nectarine

BELLY BENEFIT
Opt for ricotta over mozzarella to trim 200 calories and 11g saturated fat. Yes, you're welcome.
TOTAL 200 CALORIES

5 DINNER
CHICKEN KEBABS

- 150g chicken breast, cubed
- ½ red pepper, cut in squares
- ½ onion, cut in squares
- 2 portobello mushrooms, cut in squares
- 1 tbsp light olive oil

BELLY BENEFIT
Brush your kebabs with olive oil to cut post-dinner cravings. Unlike other oils, it sends signals to your brain to tell it to stop eating. Helpful.
TOTAL 350 CALORIES

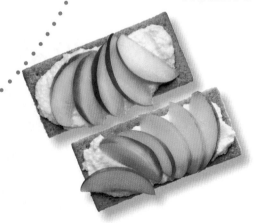

WORDS: AMELIA JEAN JONES AND KERI GLASSMAN. PHOTOGRAPHY: LEVI BROWN

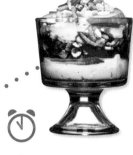

1 BREAKFAST
PANCAKES WITH ALMOND BUTTER AND BERRIES

- 2 wholewheat pancakes
- 1 tbsp almond butter
- 20g each of blackberries, blueberries and raspberries

BELLY BENEFIT
Almond butter keeps blood sugar steady, a study in *Nutrition & Metabolism* found. So you're less likely to nip to Greggs for a pre-lunch sugar hit.

TOTAL 310 CALORIES

2 SNACK
PEACH AND OAT CRUNCH POT

- 110g non-fat Greek yoghurt
- 1 small peach, sliced
- 15g Special K Oats & Honey

BELLY BENEFIT
Yoghurt revs your body's fat-burning engines, according to a study in the *International Journal Of Obesity*.

TOTAL 260 CALORIES

Week 1: Sunday

How about a berry-filled breakfast in bed, smoked salmon in the afternoon and a slap-up roast in the evening? Welcome to your flat belly Sunday

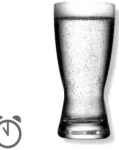

6 EXTRA SNACK
A BEER

ADD *350ml light beer (100 calories)*
SUBTRACT *The avocado from lunch and use only 2 tsp of oil at dinner (100 calories).*
TOTAL 100 CALORIES

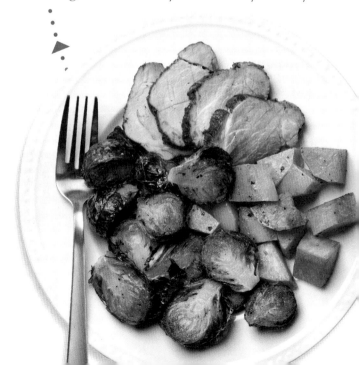

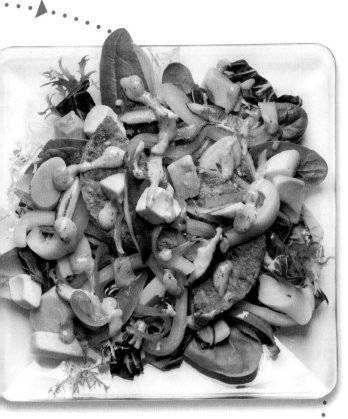

3 LUNCH
VEGGIE BURGER SALAD

- 1 cooked Linda McCartney Quarter Pounder Burger
- 140g mixed leaves
- 40g avocado, diced
- 70g hearts of palm, sliced
- 70g yellow pepper, sliced
- 80g mushrooms, sautéed
- 80g yellow onions, sautéed
- 1 tbsp Dijon mustard
- 1 tbsp olive oil
- ½ tsp salt
- ¾ tsp pepper

BELLY BENEFIT
Spoon 20g mustard onto any meal and a couple of hours later, your fat burning will have increased by up to 20%. It's thanks to its 'isothiocyanates', which increase levels of the fat-burning hormone ephedrine. Hello, hot stuff.
TOTAL: 380 CALORIES

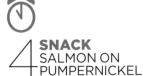

4 SNACK
SALMON ON PUMPERNICKEL

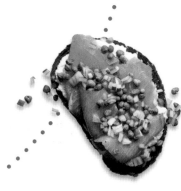

- 1 slice Biona Organic Pumpernickel Bread
- 1 tbsp non-fat cottage cheese
- 60g smoked salmon
- 2 tbsp capers
- 1½ tbsp minced onions

BELLY BENEFIT
With slow-release carbohydrates to keep energy levels stable, the pumpernickel will keep you from snacking until dinnertime.
TOTAL 150 CALORIES

5 DINNER
PORK WITH ROASTED VEGETABLES

- 90g pork tenderloin, roasted
- 200g baked butternut squash, cubed
- 300g Brussels sprouts (cooked in 1 tbsp olive oil)
- ½ tsp salt
- 1 tsp black pepper

BELLY BENEFIT
Research in the journal *Nutrition* found the zinc and vitamin B12 in pork are crucial to your body's energy regulation. Translation: no sugar slump before bedtime.
TOTAL 400 CALORIES

WORDS: AMELIA JEAN JONES AND KERI GLASSMAN. PHOTOGRAPHY: LEVI BROWN

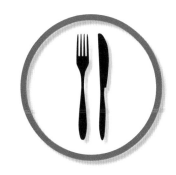

HALF WAY THERE!

Well, you've feasted on week's worth of tasty meals and snacks that have kept temptation at bay and pushed your body's fat-burning ability to the limit. By now you should be noticing a little more space around your waistband. Maybe, just maybe, you're starting to check out the result of your hard work in the mirror. Hey, it's okay. (Saucy winks are optional). Give yourself a pat on the back, and spur yourself on for the last stretch with some flat belly inspiration...

"I ate clean to get lean"

Natasha Bugg, 24, tells us how she changed her attitude to food and smashed her goal weight

Stuck down a body cul-de-sac, it took a bereavement in Natasha's family to inspire her to re-evaluate her attitude to food, exercise – and ultimately, her health.

THEN "As a chubby child, I always assumed my puppy fat would just melt away once I reached my teens, but it didn't. Later, at university, late nights, alcohol and eating lazy convenience meals meant the weight piled on even more, and I rocketed from a size 14 to 18. In my final year, I joined a gym and started making salads in an attempt to shed pounds. But in reality, going to Zumba twice a month and eating lettuce with a chicken Kiev was never going to work. When I graduated in August 2012, I was 15st 7lb."

HOW "That year, I lost my grandad – he was still quite young. I was at an emotional low and I knew I had to take

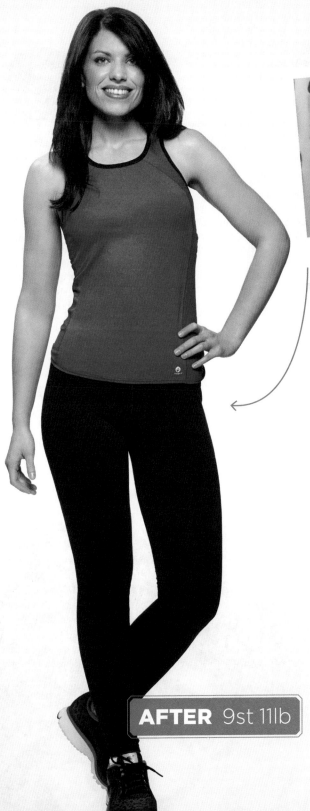

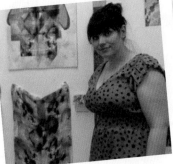

BEFORE 15st 7lb

AFTER 9st 11lb

control of my health. So I began a cleaner diet, ditching all the processed foods for the most natural ingredients I could find. Swapping my morning muffin for a handful of almonds wasn't so hard, and I actually preferred pumpkin seeds and chicken with salad to the creamy dressings and sandwich meat I'd been eating before. I went to the gym five times a week, often for up to three or four hours, to swim and do body combat classes. It sounds excessive, but it became a way to vent my emotions."

NOW "I haven't lost any more weight in the past six months, but at 9st 11lb and a size eight, I've reached my body's 'healthy' weight. And treats aren't out of the question – I have a healthy eating lifestyle rather than a diet. So if I fancy some chocolate, I'll have it, but I don't touch anything with less than 70% cocoa. I still visit the gym five times a week, but I go because I want to and I enjoy it. It's a way of life for me now."

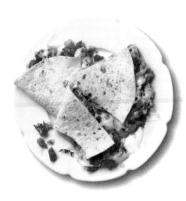

1 BREAKFAST
SCRAMBLED EGGSADILLA

- 1 whole egg
- 1 egg white
- 2 tbsp chopped green pepper
- 2 tbsp chopped red onion
- 18in whole-wheat tortilla
- 30g Cheddar cheese, grated
- 2 tbsp chunky salsa

BELLY BENEFIT
Good news! Peppers prevent new fat cells forming, thanks to a compound called piperine, which interferes with the body's fat-building genes. Now that should pep you up.
TOTAL 330 CALORIES

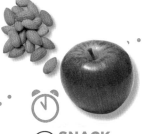

2 SNACK
APPLE AND ALMONDS

- 20 almonds
- 1 medium apple

BELLY BENEFIT
Studies have shown that ursolic acid, a compound found in apple skin, could protect us from obesity, as it increases our muscle stores.
TOTAL 230 CALORIES

Week 2: Monday

Be a prawn star with this protein packed salad lunch, crunch a bunch of antioxidants and get porky for a filling dinner. Flat belly here we come

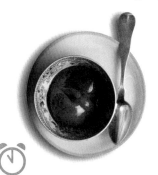

6 EXTRA SNACK
RASPBERRY SORBET TREAT

ADD 100g Rookbeare Sorbet Raspberry (£4.29, ocado.com).
SUBTRACT The potato at dinner. Sweet swapsies.

TOTAL 100 CALORIES

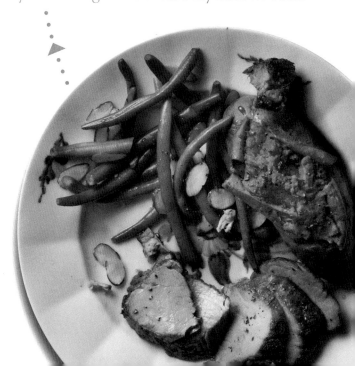

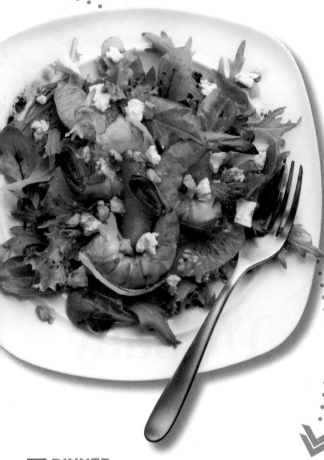

3 LUNCH
PRAWN SPRING SALAD

- 1½ tsp olive oil
- 1 tbsp balsamic vinegar
- 2 tsp lemon juice
- 70g mixed leaves
- 100g cooked prawns
- 30g goat's cheese
- 60g orange segments
- 1 tbsp chopped walnuts

BELLY BENEFIT
Minus the chips, the acetic acid in vinegar suppresses the building of body fat by increasing the temperature of your liver. Now that's hot stuff.
TOTAL 390 CALORIES

4 SNACK
RED PEPPER CRUDITÉS

- 120g roasted red peppers
- 35g crumbled feta
- 1 tsp crushed garlic
- ½ tsp olive oil
- 180g broccoli and carrot

BELLY BENEFIT
Vitamin K in broccoli keeps your insulin in check. Translation: you're more likely to burn fat than store it. Dip away.
TOTAL 180 CALORIES

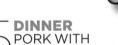

5 DINNER
PORK WITH SWEET POTATO

- 115g pork tenderloin
- 125g steamed green beans
- 2 tbsp sliced almonds
- 1 baked sweet potato

BELLY BENEFIT
Pound for pound, a lean pork tenderloin has less fat than a chicken breast. It's also high in niacin and selenium (nutrients more commonly associated with red meat), which help you grow muscle. Your roast can get you ripped.
TOTAL 370 CALORIES

WORDS: AMELIA JEAN JONES AND KERI GLASSMAN. PHOTOGRAPHY: LEVI BROWN

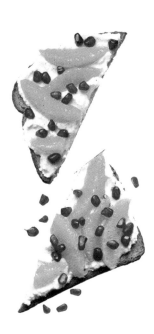

1 BREAKFAST
ORANGE AND POMEGRANATE RICOTTA TOAST

- 60g low-fat ricotta cheese mixed with 2 tsp honey
- 1 slice wholemeal toast
- 1 navel orange
- 1 tbsp pomegranate seeds
- ¾ tsp nutmeg

BELLY BENEFIT
Studies show these ruby-red seeds help cut body fat and increase metabolism. Sweet.
TOTAL 290 CALORIES

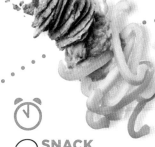

2 SNACK
GUAC-PEPPER CRUNCH

- 5 Nairn's Oat Cracker Thins
- 85g reduced-fat guacamole
- 12 strips yellow pepper

BELLY BENEFIT
Avocado contains healthy fats that curb pre-lunch snack urges.
TOTAL 260 CALORIES

Week 2: Tuesday

Captain Crunch or smooth operator? Both. A variety of textures will help keep your tastebuds on side and deliver you the nutrients you need

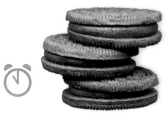

6 EXTRA SNACK
OREOS

ADD 3 Chocolate Creme Oreo biscuits
SUBTRACT Feta from lunch and four crackers from your morning snack
TOTAL 225 CALORIES

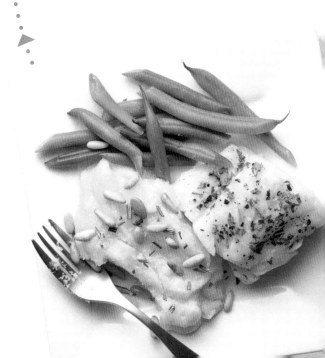

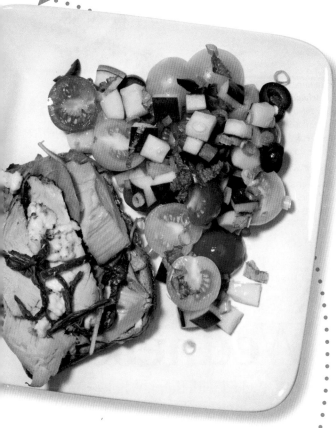

WORDS: AMELIA JEAN JONES AND KERI GLASSMAN. PHOTOGRAPHY: LEVI BROWN.

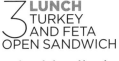

3 LUNCH
TURKEY AND FETA OPEN SANDWICH

- 1 slice wholemeal bread
- 85g sliced turkey breast
- 60g baby spinach
- 60g sun-dried tomatoes
- 30g feta cheese
- 12 yellow or red cherry tomatoes, halved
- 60g chopped cucumber
- 4 black olives, chopped
- 1 tbsp chopped spring onion
- ½ tsp lemon juice
- 1 tsp fresh mint

BELLY BENEFIT
Top bread with turkey, spinach, sun-dried tomatoes and feta cheese. Pop under the grill for 6 minutes, or until golden. Serve with salad. Enjoy!
TOTAL 420 CALORIES

4 SNACK
CINNANUT-TOPPED SWEET POTATO

- 1 medium sweet potato, baked
- 2 tbsp non-fat Greek yoghurt
- ½ tsp cinnamon
- 1 tbsp chopped pecans

BELLY BENEFIT
Eating 3-5 grams of fat with sweet potato prevents oxidative damage from strenuous exercise so you can work out for longer.
TOTAL 180 CALORIES

5 DINNER
STEAMED COD WITH GREEN BEANS AND POLENTA

- 85g cod
- 1 tsp chopped fresh parsley
- Pinch of salt
- Pinch of pepper
- 60g dry polenta
- 60ml skimmed milk
- 1 tbsp pine nuts
- ½ tsp rosemary
- 120g cooked green beans

BELLY BENEFIT
Steam the cod for 6 minutes and cook the polenta with milk. Top with pine nuts, rosemary and green beans before seasoning. Rosemary's carnosic acid helps reduce weight gain. Tasty.
TOTAL 350 CALORIES

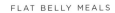

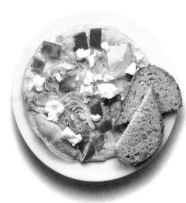

1 BREAKFAST
TOMATO, FETA AND ARTICHOKE FRITTATA

- 1 egg
- 1 egg white
- Olive oil spray
- 40g chopped tomatoes
- 40g canned artichoke hearts, drained and chopped
- 1 tsp chopped shallot
- 3 tbsp crumbled feta
- 1 slice wholegrain bread, toasted

BELLY BENEFIT
Eating wholegrains can reduce inflammation and help cut belly flab. No grain, no gain.
TOTAL 290 CALORIES

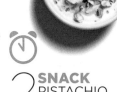

2 SNACK
PISTACHIO YOGHURT

- 150g non-fat Greek yoghurt
- 20 shelled pistachios
- 1 tsp honey

BELLY BENEFIT
According to the journal *Obesity*, eating nuts twice a week helps stave off weight gain.
TOTAL 180 CALORIES

Week 2: Wednesday

Fibre? Check. Omega-3? Got it. B vits? Packed with them. Wholegrains, nuts and seeds sneak some powerful fat-torching goodies into today's meals

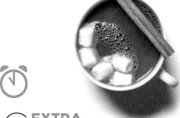

6 EXTRA SNACK
ALMOND HOT CHOCOLATE

ADD *Cocoa. Mix 250ml hot unsweeted almond milk with 1½ tbsp sugar and 2 tsp unsweetened cocoa. Serve with 5 mini marshmallows (18 calories) and a cinnamon stick.* **SUBTRACT** *The feta at breakfast.*
TOTAL 125 CALORIES

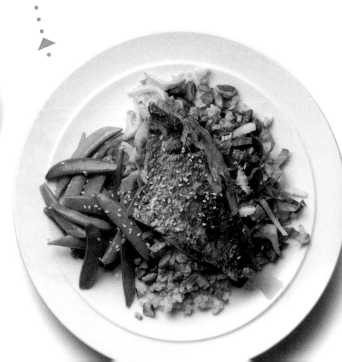

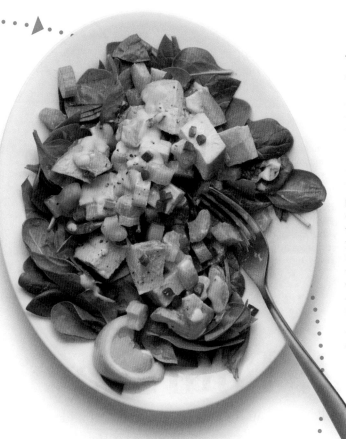

3 LUNCH
GREEN SPICY CHICKEN SALAD

- *150g roasted skinless chicken breast, cubed*
- *1 tbsp fresh lemon juice*
- *4 tsp Dijon mustard*
- *½ chilli, diced*
- *½ medium celery stalk, chopped*
- *30g baby spinach*
- *Black pepper*

BELLY BENEFIT
Chop fresh chillies into any dish to encourage thermogenesis – your body's heat-generating response – which helps burn calories. "For maximum effect, eat chilli-based foods daily," says Jeya Henry, professor of human nutrition at Oxford Brookes University. Not an excuse to have The Raj on speed dial, mind.
TOTAL 260 CALORIES

5 DINNER
ASIAN SNAPPER

- *30g raw pistachios*
- *30g cooked millet*
- *20g bok choi*
- *170g cooked snapper*
- *4tsp low-sodium soy sauce*
- *2 tsp sesame seeds*
- *100g sugar snap peas, cooked*

BELLY BENEFIT
Millet isn't just for the birds – it's incredibly high in fibre and can stave off an appetite attack with little difficulty. Along with the snapper, it will deliver a double dose of vitamin B12 to your metabolism.
TOTAL 540 CALORIES

4 SNACK
TOMATO AND MOZZARELLA

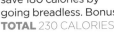

- *2 medium tomatoes, sliced*
- *60g low-fat mozzarella*
- *1 tsp olive oil*
- *1 tsp fresh oregano*
- *1½ tbsp minced onions*

BELLY BENEFIT
Think of it as bruschetta, but better for you. You save 180 calories by going breadless. Bonus!
TOTAL 230 CALORIES

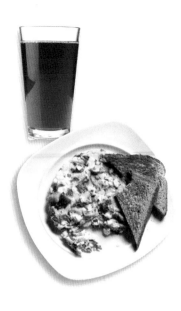

1 BREAKFAST
MUSHROOM AND FETA FRITTATA

- 2 egg whites
- 1 whole egg
- 15g fresh spinach
- 55g chopped mushrooms
- 30g feta cheese
- 1 tsp fresh coriander
- 1 slice oat-bran bread
- 60ml pomegranate juice mixed with 170ml water

BELLY BENEFIT
Researchers at Queen Margaret University found that pomegranate juice can suppress appetite.
TOTAL 350 CALORIES

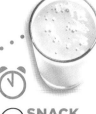

2 SNACK
PEACH SMOOTHIE

- 1 tbsp Meridian Sunflower Seed Butter
- 110g non-fat Greek yoghurt
- 1 small peach

BELLY BENEFIT
Sunflower seed butter has the protein of peanut, but a third less sat fat.
TOTAL 200 CALORIES

Week 2: Thursday

Get green today. Your body will be so grateful for the fibre and antioxidants in the spinach, kale and broccoli it'll burn even more fat to say thank you

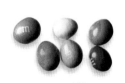

6 EXTRA SNACK
M&M TREAT

ADD *Packet fun-size Peanut M&M's*
SUBTRACT *Half the feta at breakfast and the beef dressing. Done deal!*
TOTAL 90 CALORIES

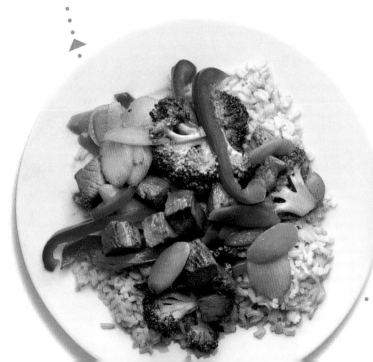

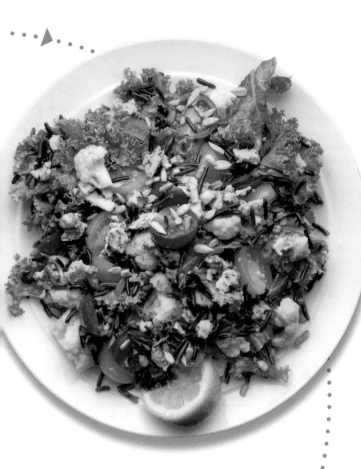

3 LUNCH
WILD RICE, CAULIFLOWER AND KALE SALAD

- 40g cooked wild rice
- 70g kale, chopped
- 50g cauliflower florets
- 150g cherry tomatoes
- 2 tbsp sunflower seeds
- 30g crumbled blue cheese
- 2 tsp olive oil
- 1½ tsp lemon juice

BELLY BENEFIT
Three cauliflower servings a week improves liver function, which, in turn, helps you burn fat, says the University of Hawaii. A whole bunch of goodness.
TOTAL 330 CALORIES

4 SNACK
CRACKERS AND AVOCADO

- 1 pack of Ryvita Sweet Chilli Minis
- 50g guacamole
- 80g sliced apple

BELLY BENEFIT
Pectin in apples limits the fat our cells can absorb, a Florida State University study found. One a day it is.
TOTAL 220 CALORIES

5 DINNER
TERIYAKI BEEF AND VEG STIR-FRY

- 90g beef tenderloin, cubed
- 2 tbsp reduced-salt teriyaki sauce
- 3 tbsp light honey and mustard dressing
- 32g sliced carrots
- 50g chopped broccoli
- 35g sliced water chestnuts
- 40g sliced peppers
- 100g cooked brown rice

BELLY BENEFIT
Choose grass-fed beef. Meat from cattle that graze on grass has higher levels of conjugated linoleic acid, which can help reduce body fat.
TOTAL 400 CALORIES

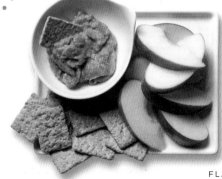

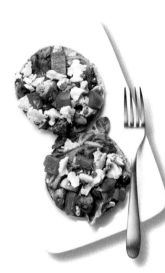

1 BREAKFAST
TOFU PEPPER SCRAMBLE

- 1 tsp olive oil
- 110g soft tofu, crumbled
- 1 red pepper, chopped
- 80g baby portobello mushrooms
- 30g spinach, chopped
- 28g reduced-fat mozzarella
- 1 tsp oregano
- 1 Warburtons Soft Brown Sandwich Thin

BELLY BENEFIT
Swapping eggs for tofu is a great way to get calcium. Sauté the tofu and veg for 5-7 minutes, top with the cheese and oregano and serve on the toasted Sandwich Thin.
TOTAL 328 CALORIES

2 SNACK
ALMOND APPLES

- 1 large apple, sliced
- 2 tsp almond butter
- 1 tsp cinnamon

BELLY BENEFIT
A recent UK study found dieters given cinnamon pills lost 300% more abdominal fat than those given a placebo.
TOTAL 187 CALORIES

Week 2: Friday

Keep going all day – and well into the evening if need be – with today's appetite slaying mix of filling protein and fibre-rich fruit and veg

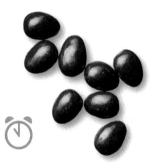

6 EXTRA SNACK
CHOC RAISINS

- Handful (30g) Thorntons Chocolate Smothered Raisins

HAVE THIS IF...
You've exercised for at least 30 minutes today.
TOTAL 120 CALORIES

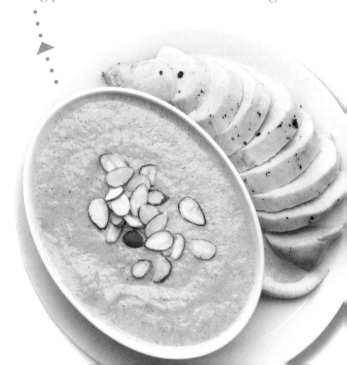

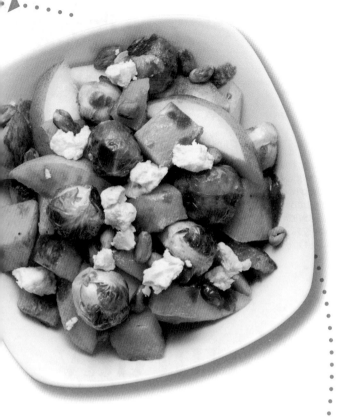

3 LUNCH
ROAST PUMPKIN AND PEAR SALAD

- 150g pumpkin, cubed
- 2 tsp olive oil
- 75g Brussels sprouts
- 28g goat's cheese
- 2 tbsp pistachios
- 1 medium pear, sliced
- 2 tbsp balsamic vinegar
- 2 tsp mustard

BELLY BENEFIT
Pumpkin is full of potassium, which banishes bloating by drawing water into your body's cells. The result: a flatter tum. Plus, its natural sweetness helps satisfy sugar cravings. Roast it in the oil with the sprouts for 30 minutes, then mix in the other ingredients.
TOTAL 387 CALORIES

4 SNACK
CAULI-CHEESE BITES

- 100g cauliflower florets
- 1 tbsp olive oil
- 3 tbsp grated Parmesan
- Salt and pepper, to taste

BELLY BENEFIT
Cauliflower is rich in phytochemicals, diet-friendly substances that stimulate metabolism to burn belly fat.
TOTAL 238 CALORIES

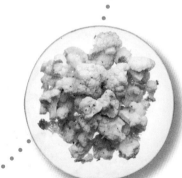

5 DINNER
LEMON CHICKEN WITH CHEESY BROCCOLI SOUP

- 100g broccoli, chopped
- 150g parsnips, chopped
- 180ml chicken stock
- 20g reduced-fat grated Cheddar cheese
- 1 tbsp sliced almonds
- 100g chicken breast
- 1 tsp lemon juice

BELLY BENEFIT
Steam the vegetables then blend with the stock, cheese and nuts. Serve with the chicken, baked and drizzled with the lemon.
TOTAL 360 CALORIES

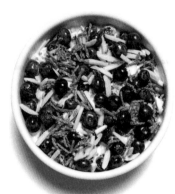

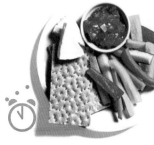

1 BREAKFAST
ALMOND BERRY CEREAL

- 30g Kellogg's All-Bran Original
- 75g blueberries
- 2 tbsps slivered almonds
- 1 tbsp ground flaxseed
- 250ml fat-free milk

BELLY BENEFIT
Pimping your cereal has serious slimming rewards: the healthy omega-3 fats in flaxseeds prolong satiety, according to a study in *Appetite*. The blueberries also keep you full, providing 5 per cent of your daily fibre needs.
TOTAL 360 CALORIES

2 SNACK
CHILLI CHEESE CRUDITÉS

- 2 Ryvita crackers
- 150g raw carrots, peppers and cucumbers
- 2 wedges Laughing Cow Light cheese
- 2 tbsp salsa

BELLY BENEFIT
Chilli has been found to speed your metabolism for hours after eating it*.
TOTAL 185 CALORIES

Week 2: Saturday

Omega-3 is your fat belly best friend. Let it come out to play with seeds and oily fish. And if you can get to the gym there's a reward for you

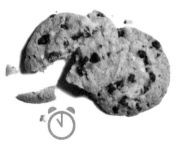

6 EXTRA SNACK
COOKIE

- 2 Maryland Choc Chip biscuits

HAVE THIS IF...
You've exercised for at least 30 minutes today.
TOTAL 135 CALORIES

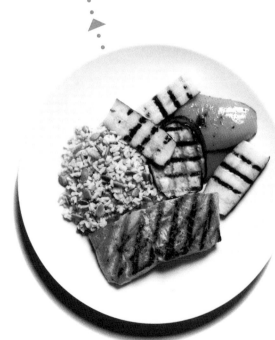

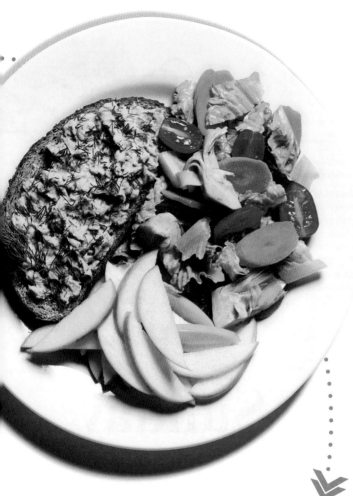

3 LUNCH TUNA SALAD SANDWICH

- 85g tinned tuna
- 1 tsp Dijon mustard
- 1 tbsp plain low-fat yoghurt
- ¼ tsp dill
- 1 slice wholegrain bread
- Handful of cos lettuce, chopped
- 40g sliced carrot
- 40g cherry tomatoes
- 40g artichoke hearts, quartered
- 1 tsp olive oil
- 1 small Granny Smith apple, sliced

BELLY BENEFIT
Wholegrain bread helps you in two ways: the fibre fills you up, and studies have found a diet rich in whole grains is associated with a lower BMI and a smaller waist circumference.
TOTAL 355 CALORIES

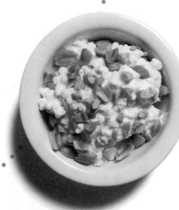

4 SNACK COTTAGE CHEESE

- 150g low-fat cottage cheese
- 1 tbsp unsalted peanuts

BELLY BENEFIT
Snack on dairy whenever you can; consuming 1,800mg of calcium a day can block the absorption of about 80 calories, according to a University of Tennessee study.
TOTAL 140 CALORIES

5 DINNER SALMON WITH VEGGIES

- 115g grilled salmon
- 150g grilled vegetables (courgette, aubergine and peppers)
- 90g cooked brown rice
- 1 tbsp pumpkin seeds

BELLY BENEFIT
Pumpkin seeds are a rich source of monounsaturated fats, which research in *Diabetes Care* has found can help reduce fat – specifically around the stomach.
TOTAL 460 CALORIES

PHOTOGRAPHY: JEFF HARRIS. · SOURCE: PHYSIOLOGY & BEHAVIOR

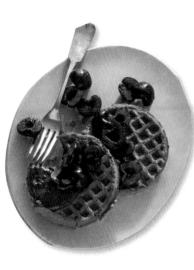

1 BREAKFAST
CHERRY WAFFLES

- 154g pitted fresh cherries
- 2 home-made wholegrain waffles
- 1 tbsp almond butter
- 10g melted dark chocolate

BELLY BENEFIT
The red anthocyanin pigment in cherries boosts the enzymes that oxidise fat, while also nixing muscle pain post-gym. Time to pop yours.
TOTAL 350 CALORIES

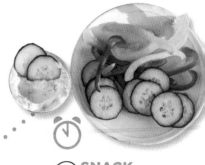

2 SNACK
CRUDITÉS AND DILL DIP

- 1 tsp chopped fresh dill
- 1 tsp olive oil
- 100g sliced cucumber
- 90g sliced peppers
- 100g non-fat Greek yoghurt

BELLY BENEFIT
The protein osteocalcin, found in olive oil, can help shed visceral fat.
TOTAL 130 CALORIES

Week 2: Sunday

Waffle away this morning with a antioxidant-loaded breakfast, then treat yourself to burger and ice cream the flat belly way

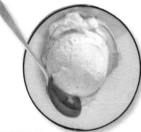

6 EXTRA SNACK
GOAT'S MILK ICE CREAM

ADD 100g St Helen's Farm Vanilla Goat's Milk Ice Cream, drizzled with 1 tsp olive oil and sprinkled with salt.

SUBTRACT 1 waffle from breakfast (85 calories) and the bun from lunch (80 calories).
TOTAL 165 CALORIES

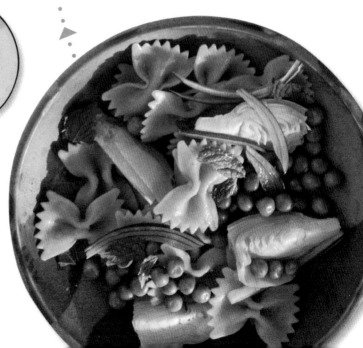

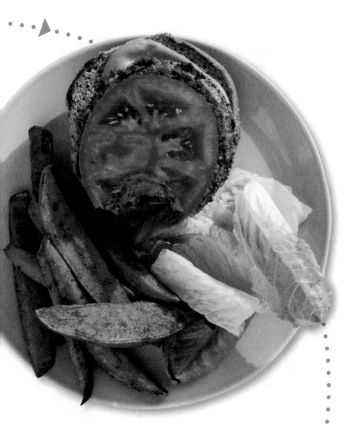

3 LUNCH
VEGGIE BURGER WITH FRIES

- *1 vegetarian quarter pounder burger*
- *½ wholemeal burger bun*
- *2 leaves romaine lettuce*
- *1 thick slice tomato*
- *2 tsp Dijon mustard*
- *1 small sweet potato*
- *1 tsp olive oil*
- *Cumin, cinnamon and paprika to season*

BELLY BENEFIT
Studies show just 1 tsp hot mustard can boost your metabolism by 20 per cent – so spice up your life and your lunch.
TOTAL 480 CALORIES

4 SNACK
ORANGES AND CASHEWS

- *2 small oranges*
- *15g cashews*

BELLY BENEFIT
The natural sugars in OJ turbocharge metabolism by up to 25 per cent, so you'll burn more of the calories you eat later. Juicy.
TOTAL 180 CALORIES

5 DINNER
SUMMER PEA AND MINT PASTA

- *60g wholegrain farfalle pasta*
- *1 tsp olive oil*
- *80g artichoke hearts*
- *30g sliced red onion*
- *10 asparagus spears*
- *25g peas*
- *1 tbsp chopped fresh mint*

BELLY BENEFIT
Humble peas are a rich source of zinc, which boosts levels of leptin – a hormone that alerts your brain when your stomach has had enough. Hap-pea tummy.
TOTAL 360 CALORIES

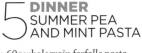

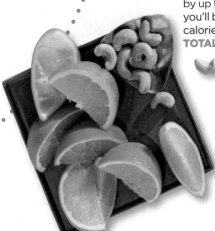

PHOTOGRAPHY: JEFF HARRIS.

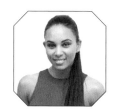

MY FLAT BELLY DIARY:

Louise Hazel

How does a former Commonwealth champion heptathlete stay in shape in retirement? If you're Louise Hazel, you readjust your diet

- -

MONDAY

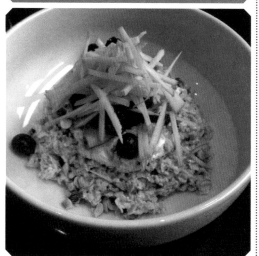

7:30am
Bircher muesli

11am
Apple, handful of mixed nuts

1:30pm
2 scrambled eggs on rye toast

3pm
Green smoothie

7pm
Chicken escalope, hash brown and kale

8pm
Green tea

I've been very aware of my body since I retired from competing. For example, I ended up gaining five pounds when I stopped training. My whole diet has changed now. I base all my meals on protein and have also cut down on the carb content.

TUESDAY

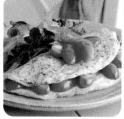

7am
Yoghurt, seeds and berries

10:30am
Pear, handful of walnuts

2pm
Tomato omelette

2:30pm
Beetroot juice

7:30pm
Lamb stew with cous cous

8pm
Chai tea

With the change in my diet came a drop in energy levels. I eat low-GI foods, such as beetroot and walnuts, every three hours to keep my blood-sugar levels constant.

WEDNESDAY

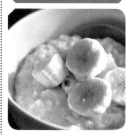

8am
Porridge and half a banana

11am
Seeds and berries

1:30pm
2 eggs with smoked salmon

3pm
Popcorn with almond butter

7pm
Steak, potatoes and kale

7:30pm
Peppermint tea

I have colitis, a bowel condition, so I try not to eat foods that stress out my system. Since I cut out dairy recently, I'm less bloated and have more energy. I wish I'd done it years ago.

AS TOLD TO: AMELIA JEAN JONES. PHOTOGRAPHY: GETTY IMAGES, LOUISE HAZEL IS FOUNDER OF THE PODIUM EFFECT, THEPODIUMEFFECT.COM

THURSDAY	FRIDAY	SATURDAY	SUNDAY

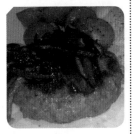 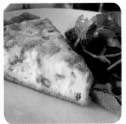 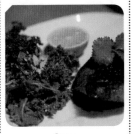 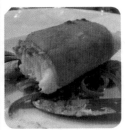

THURSDAY	FRIDAY	SATURDAY	SUNDAY
8am *Bircher muesli*	**7:30am** *Yoghurt, seeds and berries*	**9am** *Bircher muesli*	**10am** *Porridge*
10:30am *Pear, handful of walnuts*	**10am** *Apple, handful of mixed nuts*	**11am** *Seeds and berries*	**11am** *Yoghurt with passion fruit*
1pm *Tomato omelette*	**3pm** *Quiche Lorraine and salad*	**2:30pm** *2 scrambled eggs with bacon and tomatoes*	**2pm** *2 scrambled eggs and bacon*
2pm *Beetroot juice*	**4pm** *Green smoothie*	**3pm** *Green smoothie*	**3pm** *Beetroot juice*
7pm *Steak haché with tomato and couscous*	**8pm** *Black cod with edamame*	**8pm** *Steak with kale and red wine*	**7pm** *Curried cod with mashed sweet potato*
8pm *Green tea*	**9pm** *Chai tea*	**9:30pm** *Chai tea*	**8pm** *Peppermint tea*

I still train six days a week – 30 minutes running and 40 minutes of body-weight exercises. Even though I'm not training professionally I still need effective fuel.

I eat fish at least three times weekly. It has omega-3, which helps to prevent inflammatory diseases. I take a multivitamin, but it's better to get omegas from food.

I eat out about four times a week and love red wine with red meat – but I'll only have two glasses. A beetroot, apple and blueberry juice works if I'm flagging the day after.

I try to eat as healthily as I can for 95% of the time, but that 5% when I treat myself – I go all out. I will never turn down a sticky toffee pudding if you're offering!

THE EXPERT VERDICT

Our nutritionist Dr Christy Fergusson gives her feedback: "Louise eats often throughout the day, combining a mixture of good-quality protein, low glycaemic-load carbohydrates and essential fatty acids, which is the key for balancing blood-sugar levels when you're eating less than you're used to.

"I love the afternoon cleansing juices. They're a great way to add nutrients to your blood without hugely upping your calorie intake. Adding raw vegan protein powders to them, such as hemp, would keep the protein content high.

"Switching to quinoa or buckwheat over rye bread could help her colitis because they contain immunity-strengthening protein and minerals.

"Louise's diet is also very varied, which is great for reducing food intolerances – if you eat challenging foods such as dairy, meat and grains too often, your body can develop a reaction to them. Overall, I'd give her at least a silver medal!"

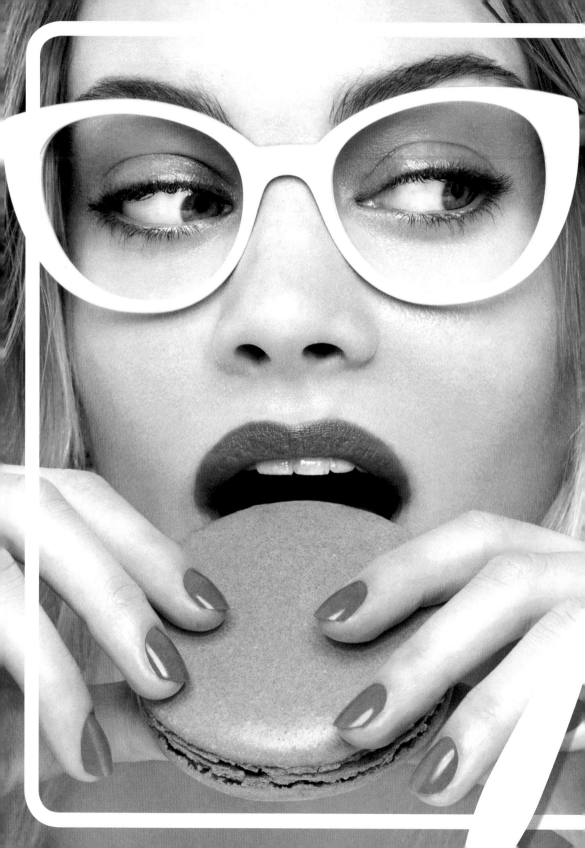

THINK YOURSELF SLIM

Losing weight isn't just about what you put in your stomach – it's also about what goes on in your head. The psychology of weight-loss is a lot more complicated than 'eat better, lose weight'. This chapter looks at how to change how you think about food and understand *why* you're eating – a vital step to keeping your new body for good.

Show your bad food habits who's boss

Certain snacks can trigger a destructive return to unhealthy behaviours. Learn how to outsmart these sneaky culprits and watch your body snap back into shape

It's a common slipup: after weeks of eating well, you're on track to lose those last five pounds. You deserve a reward. But fast-forward 30 minutes and the scene looks like feeding time at London Zoo.

In the same way that some drugs pave the way for even harder ones, a weakness for a certain food can open the door to an avalanche of bad eating choices, says Gary Wenk, author of *Your Brain on Food*. "Some foods are like gateway drugs," he says. "From your brain's viewpoint, there is no difference." These so-called gateway foods make you feel out of control, in part because of their addictive effect on your mind and body. But fad food rehab is probably easier than you think.

Here's how it works: merely looking at or thinking about a food you love switches on the reward region of your brain, the nucleus accumbens – the same area stimulated by drugs and alcohol. This triggers a surge of dopamine, the feelgood chemical that enhances your awareness of that food (like we needed to remind you).

An Australian study found that thinking about a craving uses up so much mental energy that you can struggle to do anything else. Next time you find yourself reaching for another Hobnob, distract yourself with the Draw Something game app (free) – all you'll crave is victory.

Research also shows the more food-related words and images we are exposed to, the hungrier we get. So instead of taking your usual lunch route past Pret A Manger and Greggs, head in a direction that offers fewer temptations.

JUNK FOOD JUNKIES

Once you've taken the first bite of that treat you've been dreaming about all day, watch out. Tasting food engages all your senses. Your nervous system responds by releasing insulin, making your blood glucose levels drop and relaxing your stomach muscles, so you feel as though you need to eat more to be satisfied, says Susan Roberts, a professor of nutrition at Tufts University and co-author of *The 'I' Diet*. The result: a major binge. Of course,

---

FOODS THAT MAKE YOU DO GOOD THINGS...

Fill up with these heavenly treats to tame your appetite

Eat grapefruit, lose weight	**Embrace (good) fat to tame fat**	**Curb cravings with carbs**	**Slash pounds with protein**
Research found those who ate a grapefruit with meals lost 3.6lb in three months.	Oleic acid, found in olive oil and nuts, triggers hunger-quashing signals.	Slow-digesting starches such as spuds slay hunger. Try potato salad.	Aim for 30g protein at brekkie – two eggs and a tub of plain yoghurt.

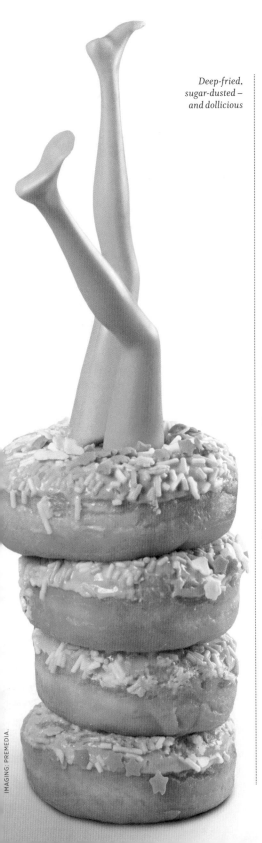

Deep-fried, sugar-dusted – and dollicious

there's a reason those cravings are almost always for fatty or sugary foods and not, say, lettuce. "The saturated fats in foods like bacon and cheese impair your brain's normal ability to regulate appetite and cravings, so you don't realise you're full until you're completely stuffed," says Kelly McGonigal, a health psychologist at Stanford University and author of *The Willpower Instinct*. "That effect on your appetite can last for up to three days, the length of time it takes your system to flush fats. So one indulgence can end up triggering a massive relapse."

APPETITE FOR DESTRUCTION

High-sugar foods increase your levels of ghrelin, a hormone that stimulates appetite and increases cravings. "So you may tell yourself 'just one bite' but find yourself wanting more," says McGonigal. 'Low-fat' foods won't help. To compensate for the lack of fat – and flavour – they're usually

Your brain has evolved to give you a high when you eat sugar

high in sugar. Anything with more than 15g of sugar per 100g is at the upper end (a low-sugar food is 5g or less per 100g).

Sugar has been shown to enhance memory storage, which may explain why you want it. Your brain has evolved to give you a high when you eat sugar. "The brain responds to both sugar and fat by releasing endorphins," says Wenk. When examined chemically, those feel-good compounds are similar to morphine in their effects and can have the same kind of biological impact – which is why you wind up so desperate for a bad food fix. So just say no: quit the habit today and your body will thank you for it **WH**

IMAGING: PREMEDIA.

Willpower 2.0

Finally! We've located your willpower. FYI, it's hiding in your frontal lobe...
And needs to be exercised like a muscle. Here's how to tame that beast

1 FEED IT 24/7
The brain needs glucose to function, says Roy Baumeister, co-author of *Willpower: Rediscovering The Greatest Human Strength*. Studies show, people with steady glucose levels are more persistent at attempting an unsolvable task than those whose levels have declined. "The benefits last longer with glucose that's from protein," says Baumeister. Eat seaweed – it has as much protein as eggs, but no cholesterol. No need to forage at the beach, try Itsu Crispy Seaweed Thins (£1.00, waitrose.com).

2 CELEBRATE WISELY
Scientists have a name for that post-gym binge: compensation. "The harder your workout, the bigger you think your compensation should be," says Timothy Church, director of the Laboratory of Preventive Medicine at the Pennington Biomedical Research Center. Take a look at womenshealthmag.co.uk for low-calorie snack ideas, or choose a non-food treat. Buy an iTunes track after your workout or enjoy a cinema outing after 10 gym visits. It's a win-win situation.

3 PLAY IT SAFE
A study in the *Journal Of Personality And Social Psychology* found people with the best self-control were those who relied on willpower less during the day. In other words, they set up their lives to minimise temptation as much as possible. Limit your snack options around the office. Studies show the less choice you have and the more 'familiar' the food (read: dull), the less likely you are to eat, says research from the University of Buffalo. Rice cakes it is then.

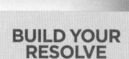

BUILD YOUR RESOLVE
Exercise your willpower with three simple rules

Meditate
It activates your prefrontal cortex (helps you make smart choices) and anterior cingulate cortex (helps you choose when to make them). Ohm.

Sit up...
...or stand tall; good posture requires mindfulness. It also builds self-confidence*, further fuelling willpower.

Speak correctly
Use full sentences, and avoid contractions and profanity. The mental effort sharpens your ability to say no.

PHOTOGRAPHY: GETTY. *SOURCES: OBESITY JOURNAL, SOCIETY FOR PERSONALITY AND SOCIAL PSYCHOLOGY, EUROPEAN JOURNAL OF SOCIAL PSYCHOLOGY

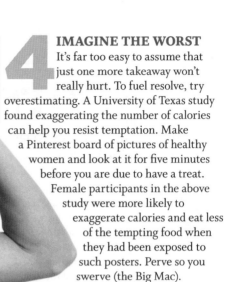

4 IMAGINE THE WORST

It's far too easy to assume that just one more takeaway won't really hurt. To fuel resolve, try overestimating. A University of Texas study found exaggerating the number of calories can help you resist temptation. Make a Pinterest board of pictures of healthy women and look at it for five minutes before you are due to have a treat. Female participants in the above study were more likely to exaggerate calories and eat less of the tempting food when they had been exposed to such posters. Perve so you swerve (the Big Mac).

5 WILL YOURSELF SLEEPY

"Willpower is lower when you're sleepy," says Kelly Glazer Baron, a clinical health psychologist. In fact, the average night owl consumes an extra 248 calories daily than someone who goes to bed earlier – with most racked up after 8pm*. Try having a glass of Biona Tart Cherry Juice (£4.69, chemistdirect.co.uk) before you head off to bed. Research from the University of Pennsylvania found tart cherries boost our melatonin levels, which helps to promote sleep. A fruity solution.

6 DELAY, DON'T DENY

Instead of saying no to food, tell yourself you'll eat later. A recent study* found that people who postponed eating crisps resisted temptation better than those who tried to refrain from having them altogether. "Postponement weakens desire at the precise time when it overwhelms willpower," says study author Dr Nicole Mead. Those pesky cravings usually last less than 10 minutes, so until it passes, make sure you keep your hands busy – paint your nails, tidy your desk. Think how much more you'll get done **WH**

She's named her guns 'Fortitude' and 'Resilience', don'tchaknow

Cheat yourself slim

Are fish and chips the key to lasting weight loss? They are if a revolutionary new scientific study is to be believed. Chip forks at the ready then…

Everyone knows how to lose weight. Fewer Crunchies, more burpees and buying something 'directional' from Issey Miyake. Problem is, it rarely sticks. So allow us to introduce a new school of scientific thought – 6:1. You stick to a healthy diet (1,500 calories) six days a week, and include one cheat strategy a week (this can be a blow-out day of 1,000 to 1,500 bad extra calories, two 500 to 750-calorie cheat meals a week or a small 150-calorie cheat daily).

Here's the scientific proof it works: participants in a study by Skidmore College in New York, over 12 weeks, had one day a week to eat whatever they liked. Even with 12 cheat days, participants cut their calories by 29 per cent and lost an average of 11 pounds. Thing was, it didn't end there; something even more interesting happened. "Many of them grew out of the free-day plan," says study author Paul Arciero. After two weeks, they were happy with one cheat meal. So what was their secret?

WIN BY LOSING

The theory goes that a diet with some kind of release valve included might just work better than one without. Countless studies show that dieters who go back to eating normally regain all if not *more* weight than they originally lost, with recent research by the University of Melbourne showing losing just five per cent of your body weight can result in chemical changes that make you crave food. To make a cheat meal *really* work, you need to be canny. Yes, you can eat a bucket of KFC if that's your thing, but if you're smart about when you actually eat it, you can trigger an even greater change.

If carbs are your thing – a massive round of toast with butter, say – try to eat them at breakfast. Research from Tel Aviv University in Israel found this lowers your ghrelin levels (the hunger hormone) for the whole day. "Just remember, some fats are essential to

> Eating carbs at brekkie lowers your hunger hormone levels for the whole day

the fat-loss process," says Jonathan White, personal trainer and fat loss expert.

"So even on your non-cheat days, do not limit foods containing omega-3 fatty acid (that's oily fish such as mackerel and salmon, flaxseed and avocado). Without this, fat loss is quickly hampered and your metabolism slows. You need to aim for around 1.5g a day." The eventual goal of this approach is what researchers call 'flexible restraint' – this is when you find yourself sticking to the plan most of the time, without forcing yourself to refuse any kind of treat.

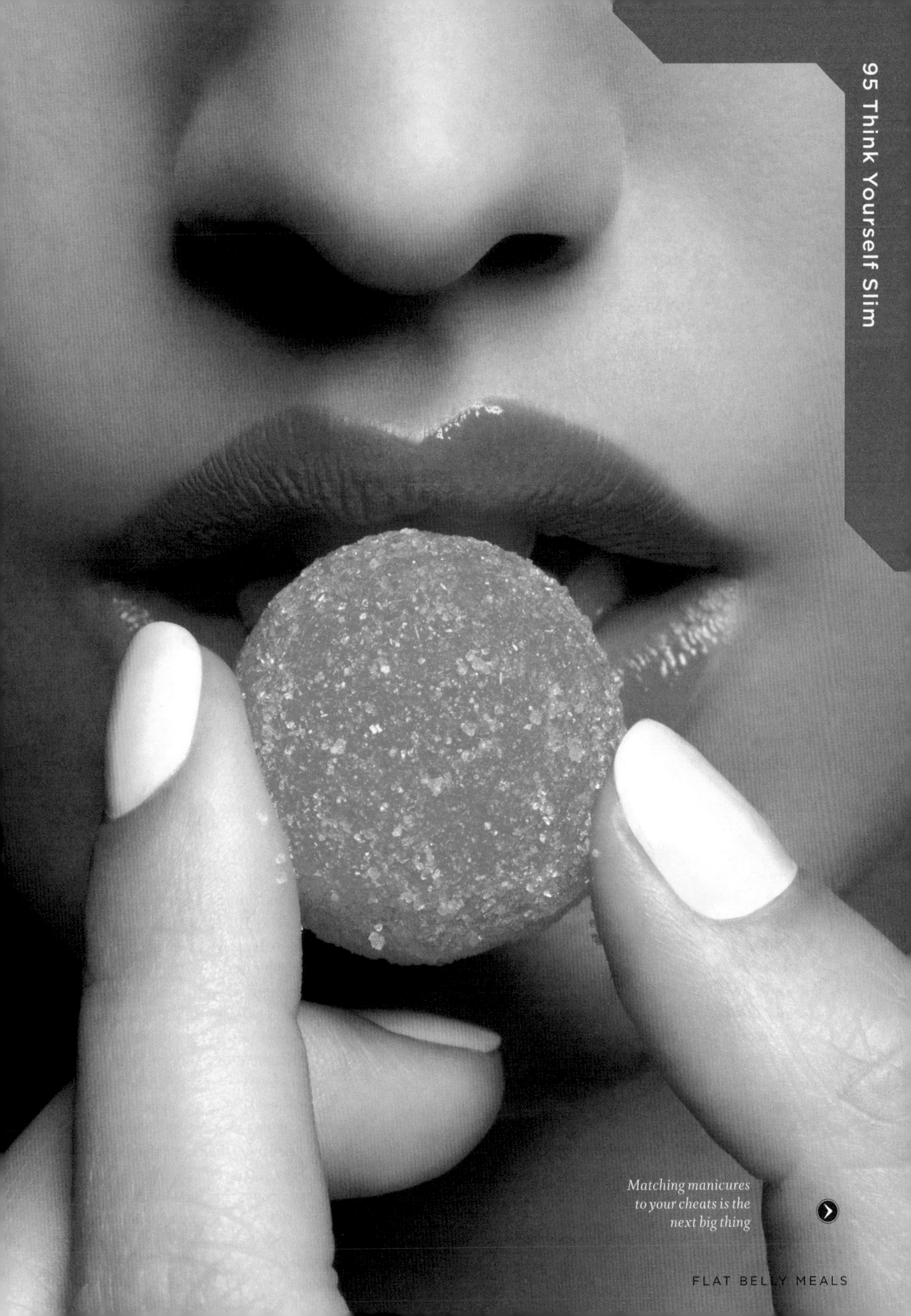

*Matching manicures
to your cheats is the
next big thing*

If you're still not convinced by this, let's stop for a moment and get more in-depth. We all know diets restrict calories and fat. What you probably don't know however is that severe fat restriction, especially that of saturated fat, has an unexpected side effect: it can lower testosterone levels. A low-carb diet could end up reducing your levels of the all-important thyroid hormone.

"Women have 5-10 per cent of the testosterone that males have," explains White. "Testosterone is essential in males *and* females as a lack of it can lead to an increased risk of depression, obesity and osteoporosis. Although women don't want to go past the 5-10 per cent figure, keeping levels steady also prevents the female hormone oestrogen from becoming overly dominant, which can lead to unwanted weight gain."

In other words, sticking religiously to a strict diet without leaving any room for cheating could result in a reduction of testosterone in your body, making it harder to retain your muscle and shed fat. While lower levels of the thyroid hormone may slow fat loss, it's also thought two other hormones could be affected – leptin, a hormone that tells you when you're full and falls when you restrict calories, while ghrelin (that pesky hunger hormone again) rises.

LET'S GET HORMONAL

Thankfully, strategic cheating could reset the hormones to optimal levels and temporarily boost your metabolism if the non-cheating part of your diet (the six days a week) cuts calories enough to give you an overall deficit. The magic number of calories is best calculated by a nutritionist using your age, weight and activity level.

You can also redress the balance by having sushi or rare steak on a couple of your non-cheat days.

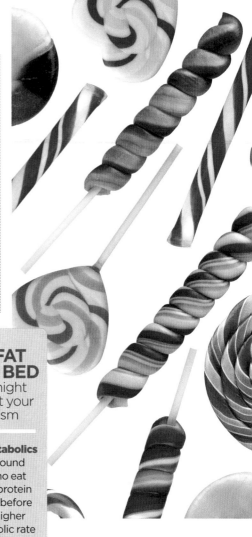

BURN FAT BEFORE BED
Eating at night could boost your metabolism

1 Speedier metabolics
A US study found fit people who eat a 150-calorie protein or carb snack before bed have a higher resting metabolic rate the next day.

2 More muscle
Drinking a protein shake before bed helps build muscle as you sleep and keeps your metabolism active in the night.

3 Baggier trousers
In a Wayne State University study, people who ate cereal before bed lost 2 pounds in a month. Those abstaining lost just half a pound.

The less the meat is cooked the more protein you absorb. A study in the *American Journal For Clinical Nutrition* found ghrelin levels fall if 60 per cent of your plate is covered by high-protein foods.

Leptin is the name of the hormone that is most affected by the cheat-day theory. Research at the University of Washington found that after a period of fasting, a 're-feed' can reset levels of the hormone to where they were before you started. For examples, good old fish and chips is the perfect cheat. The carbs in the potato

ADDITIONAL WORDS: NATALIE DYE. PHOTOGRAPHY:

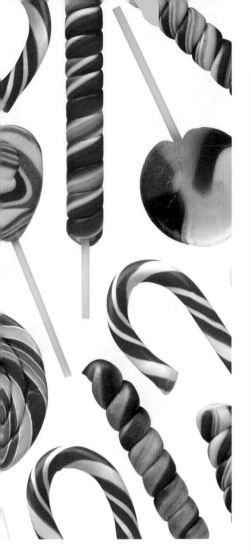

been curtailing your fat intake, you'll end up wanting a high-fat cheat – burgers and cheesecake. If you've been sticking to low-carb all this time, you're going to be desperate for pasta and pizza.

Dinner is the ideal cheat meal because it's the easiest one to monitor, whereas a weekend cheat could lead to two days worth of bingeing. "Put a time limit on your cheating, giving yourself 45 minutes to an hour," says White. "You'll eat more if the period is extended and it gives you less opportunity to dip into dessert."

On no account should you use the cheat as a reward for a fantastic workout

Another effective cheat strategy is to go for your cheat meal the night before your toughest gym session. "If chocolate is your treat, have 90 per cent of your bar before your workout," says White. The extra calories, combined with your improved mood, can make that training session more productive. But on no account should you use the cheat as a reward for a fantastic workout. "It is essential you nurture and feed your body nutrient-dense foods post workout to help it recover," warns White.

If one cheat isn't for you, use Aragon's formula – eat well 90 per cent of the time and leave 10 per cent of your calories for cheating. You have two more options then the weekly blow-out of up to 1,500 calories: two 500 to 750-calorie indulgences a week or a 100 to 150-calorie treat each day. Arciero's research points to the same conclusion. He gave participants 15 per cent 'free' calories. "The majority chose to spread out the 15 per cent over the week," he says. "It's an effective adherence strategy." The conclusion? So long rabbit food, hello Golden Arches! **WH**

will boost leptin quickly and a study by the Mayo Clinic found a fish-rich diet increases leptin sensitivity. This means that your body 'listens' to the message that you've had enough food and will, in turn, make it easier for you to resist another helping.

This leads us neatly on to the foods you should choose when allowing yourself that all-important day off. Your cheat choices should depend on what your diet is lacking, suggests sports nutritionist Alan Aragon. That's because "the psychological impact of militantly depriving yourself of food you like can sabotage your diet. It gives all the power to the food and takes the power away from the dieter," he explains. If you've

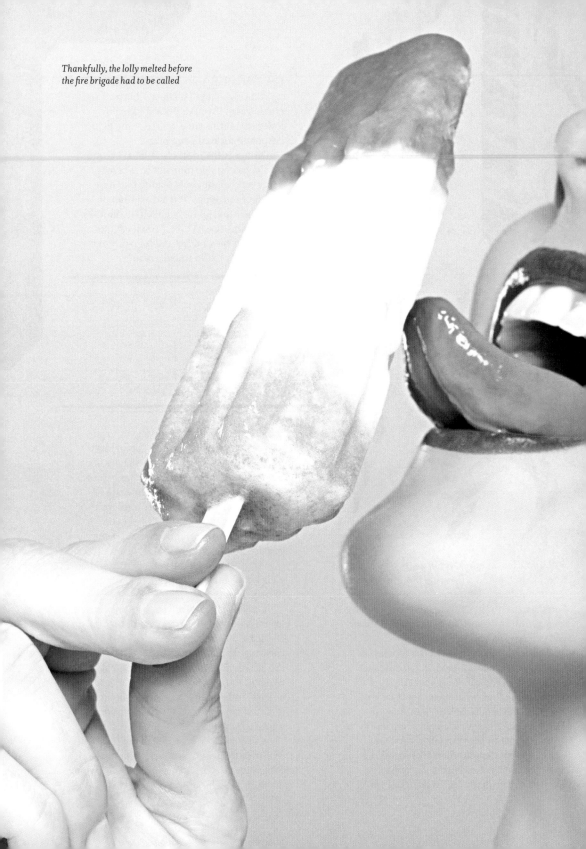

Thankfully, the lolly melted before the fire brigade had to be called

Slow down – fast food is *so* last season

When did you last take a proper lunch break? Amy Molloy finds out how you can get back in the moment – and your old jeans – with mindful eating

I knew I had a problem when, six months after buying a dining table, I realised I hadn't eaten one single meal off it. Oh, it had its uses – as a laptop desk, the perfect place to spread Sunday papers and an occasional overflow for my wardrobe. But as a place to savour a plate of food? Never. Who even sits down for 'mealtimes' anyway? I just had moveable feasts – a yoghurt on the bus to work, a sandwich scoffed over a keyboard, a bowl of pasta eaten on the sofa while watching whatever rubbish was on Film4…

And I'm not the only diner multitasking. According to a survey of British eating habits, six out of ten meals are consumed while watching television. That's if we allow ourselves to sit down long enough to watch an entire programme – the average person shovels down all three meals in a total of 23 minutes, according to the Conscious Food group, when we should be spending 20 minutes per meal for good digestion. That's some serious fast food!

The consequences of our fast-paced, unconscious way of eating are dire. Jennifer Nelson, director of clinical dietetics and nutrition at the Mayo Clinic in Minnesota, says racing to cook, eat and complete a meal puts a huge quantity of unnecessary strain on our bodies. "Side effects of speed eating include bloating and gastrointestinal problems such as nausea and diarrhoea and you're more likely to consume unwanted calories and gain weight in the long term."

A complex hormonal reaction happens between the neurotransmitters in the brain, stomach and small intestine every time we eat. Cholecystokinin is released by the intestines in response to the grub we've scoffed, then leptin (the hormone that regulates how full our stomach tells our brain we are) reacts with this to magnify how satisfied we feel. This can then trigger the brain to produce dopamine (keeping up?), our pleasure hormone, signalling how happy we are that we've eaten.

According to Harvard Medical School, the problem is that when we wolf down our chilli con carne too quickly, we don't chew it properly, preventing this complex hormonal

> According to a survey of British eating habits, six out of ten meals are consumed while watching television

response from kicking in. And it's this lack of response that can potentially result in us eating more, gaining weight – and getting no pleasure from eating, to boot. As if that wasn't bad enough, people who eat quickly have been found to be two and a half times more likely to suffer from type 2 diabetes than those who take their time, according to a paper presented at the International Congress of Endocrinology in Italy in 2012.

The good news is, it only takes a few simple strategies to reverse the damage. "Put down your knife and fork between every mouthful," says Nelson. "I also recommend patients set a timer for 20 minutes and divide their bites between that time, so meals last longer." Eating when stressed also raises the levels of cortisol in your body, which impinge digestion. Working through lunch is counterproductive if it results in an afternoon food coma.

The answer for many experts is the concept of mindful eating, which derives from Buddhist practises. Thankfully, you don't need to be able to perfect the lotus position to reap the benefits. Vietnamese monk Thich Nhat Hanh, an adviser to the Dalai Lama who wrote the book *Savor: Mindful Eating, Mindful Life*, teaches an exercise where participants are assigned 20 minutes to eat a tangerine, savouring it one segment at a time. Try it today; it's much harder than you think.

Big businesses also realise the benefits of ensuring employees take time out to eat. Harvard University School of Public Health and the California campus of Google hold silent lunch breaks, where colleagues sit around the same table but all technology use and conversation is banned. There's no escape from monitoring your mouthfuls with that one! "When we're eating, our senses should be focused on the food, not outside stimuli," says psychologist and author

OUTSMART THE ROLLER COASTER
Sidestep the top three weight-spiking times

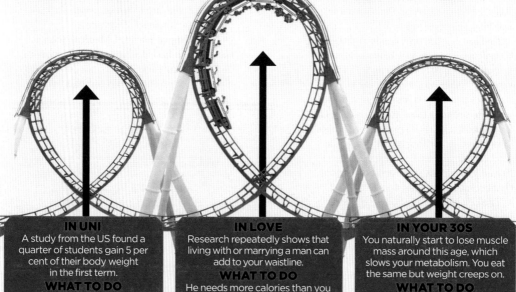

IN UNI
A study from the US found a quarter of students gain 5 per cent of their body weight in the first term.
WHAT TO DO
Have a hot lunch (think soup, not KFC). US research found aromas released by hot food make you feel full faster by affecting the satiety centres in the brain.

IN LOVE
Research repeatedly shows that living with or marrying a man can add to your waistline.
WHAT TO DO
He needs more calories than you do, so aim to eat about three-quarters of what he does. Also, make dates to do something besides eat dinner, like dancing or rockclimbing.

IN YOUR 30S
You naturally start to lose muscle mass around this age, which slows your metabolism. You eat the same but weight creeps on.
WHAT TO DO
Pump some iron to slow down the rate of loss. Two 20-to-30-minute strength training sessions a week will help keep your strong and your metabolism fired up.

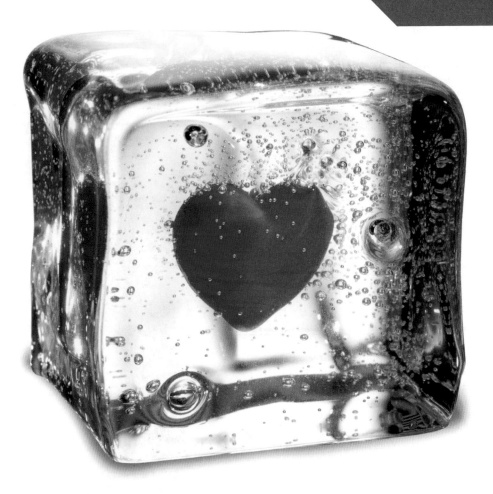

Try eating a tangerine spread out over 20 minutes; it's much harder than you think

of *Food Addiction Therapy* Kellee Waters. "We should only eat when we're hungry and stop when we're full, but sometimes we eat out of habit or because of external emotional triggers." In a recent study, 150 participants from Paris and Chicago were asked when they know a meal is over. The majority of the French subjects said when they were

"no longer hungry" or "the food no longer tastes good". But most Americans said that, for them, it was when "the plate is empty" or "the TV show we're watching has finished". Which group do you fall into?

It turns out your answer could be directly related to your waistline. A study by the University of Bristol's department of experimental psychology discovered that subjects who played solitaire while eating reported feeling less full than the group of non-distracted participants. And not only that, they also ate nearly twice as many biscuits when afternoon tea came around.

But relax, this doesn't mean to say that naughty nibbles are off the menu – just make sure you take time to think about how it feels to eat them, rather than wolf it all down and forget the pleasure ever happened: "If you ❯

do indulge in a treat, take the time to really enjoy it," says Waters. "I tell clients to take five slow deep breaths before eating anything sugary or oily. It brings us back to the present, aiding digestion and stopping us from overeating." Remember, you can always eat whenever you feel hungry. People who are

Use a proper plate and cutlery. Research shows we eat up to 30% more calories when using plastics

stuck on the idea of the standard three meals a day are far more likely to overindulge as they're aware it's not 'allowed' for them to eat again until the next window.

It helps to learn how to differentiate your emotional cravings from physical ones. Emotional cravings often manifest as a strong desire for one particular food, such as a specific brand of chocolate bar. If this is the case, try to keep yourself busy by listening to your favourite song or going for a walk. Genuine stomach hunger is generally less specific. If your body really needs fuel, then go ahead and give it what it's asking for.

Allowing yourself permission to pause isn't easy, especially in our phone-pinging 24/7 culture, so wean yourself off distractions slowly. There is no point banning all work at lunchtime if this causes you to subconsciously rush your food so you can go back to your duties. At lunchtime, if you can't leave the office, do low-tech work, such as reading a printed document or writing in a notebook.

Instead of watching television during dinner, switch on the radio and free up one of your senses. The ultimate goal is to become comfortable with eating in silence, with nothing but the food and your tastebuds' reaction to it to break the boredom. Or try

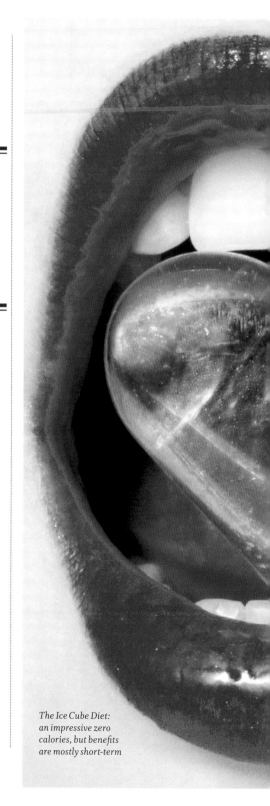

The Ice Cube Diet: an impressive zero calories, but benefits are mostly short-term

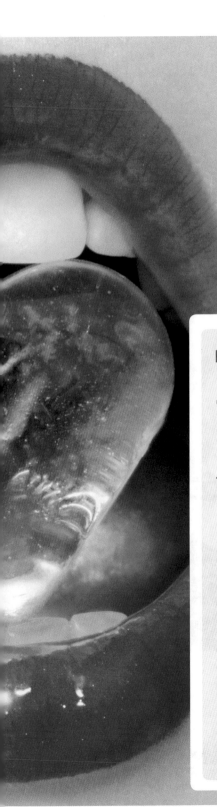

another handy strategy: use a proper plate and cutlery. In a Canadian study, participants who ate out of plastic containers while standing up went on to consume an average of 30% more calories this way.

It took a while to reset my 'chewing clock' – especially when eating with friends. My fellow diners would wolf down their meals, while I still lingered over my fourth mouthful. But the benefits were immediate. My irritable bowel syndrome quickly improved and, by stopping when I felt full, I halved my portion sizes, which meant both my dress size and food bill shrunk. Now, my dining table serves its true purpose and is my sanctuary from work deadlines. If you're reading this while eating, it's time to show your meal the respect it deserves.

HOW TO RESET YOUR EATING CLOCK

Small steps, big changes. Here are four ways to eat more mindfully... starting with tonight's dinner

1 MOVE YOUR PHONE

Keep it out of reach during meal times – books and magazines too, if you're feeling adventurous. Studies show reading while eating could increase your calorie intake by as much as 50%!

2 REGULATE AND REPEAT

Adopt some pre-dinner rituals, such as washing your hands or pausing to light a candle. It anchors the mind and, once ingrained, sends signals to your brain that you are about to eat.

3 SIT DOWN TO EAT

Canadian researchers found people who ate standing up downed 30% more calories than those who sat down because they didn't register they were eating and ate more as a result.

4 STOP THE STRETCH

Ban wearing sportswear at the meal table – elasticated clothing makes us much more likely to overeat because we're so comfortable. No more fat pants WH

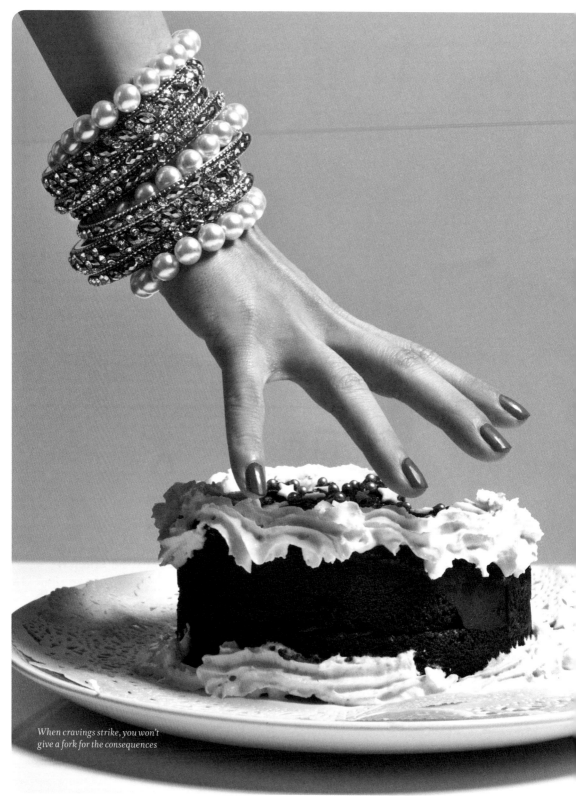

When cravings strike, you won't
give a fork for the consequences

When fat comes back

When you were a kid, yo-yoing was fun. But when it's your weight reeling up and down? Not so enjoyable. Here's how to put a stop to it – forever

Which of us hasn't high-fived ourselves for fitting into our favourite jeans again, only to have to relegate them to the back of the wardrobe a few months later? The statistics of on-again, off-again weight are pretty grim. By some estimates, 80 per cent of people who've lost weight regain every last pound, or more, after two years.

While small fluctuations on your scales are completely normal, the unhealthy behaviour that experts refer to as "weight cycling" is not. This behaviour is defined as a significant increase or decrease of body weight (generally 10 pounds or more) that occurs multiple times throughout your life.

Yo-yoing weight is not a good cycle to be in. Along with the emotional toll comes a physical one: not only is extra weight a health risk, recent studies have linked the gain-lose-gain cycle to high blood pressure, diabetes, heart disease and even cancer.

You're also more likely to end up weighing more. In an analysis of 31 long-term diet studies published in *American Psychologist*, about two-thirds of participants regained more weight than they'd initially lost: "If you go on a strict diet and gain the weight back quickly, you lose a lot of muscle and regain a lot of fat," says dietitian Dr Keith Ayoob.

METABOLIC MATHS

Experts believe a yo-yo pattern is often the result of a diet that's too restrictive, and a study reported in the journal *Obesity* backs that up. It found that people who followed a very low-calorie diet regained significantly more weight than those on a more forgiving plan. "Many women try to lose weight on crash diets with too few calories," says Dr Jude Oben, obesity consultant at Guy's & St Thomas' Hospital in London. "But I can't stress strongly enough that this quick-fix approach doesn't work. It's just not sustainable in the long term." Instead, he says, make small changes you can maintain.

Frustratingly, even on a sensible diet, your body sheds pounds reluctantly. "It's difficult to keep weight off because there is a metabolic overcompensation for weight loss," says psychologist and obesity researcher Dr Gary Foster, co-author of *Managing Obesity: A Clinical Guide*. "If you decrease

"You need to learn how to motivate yourself and override negative thoughts"

your body mass by 10 per cent, you'd expect your metabolic rate to decrease by 10 per cent, but it actually slows down more than that, by about 11 to 15 per cent."

So, why does your own metabolism thwart you? Dr Kelly Brownell, director of the Rudd Center for Food Policy and Obesity at Yale University explains: "The body may perceive dieting as a threat. It might not know the difference between Atkins and famine."

3 STEPS TO STOP YO-YOING

Build these simple habits into your life
to keep your weight steady

BECOME AWARE
Know your cues, says Dr David Kessler. That's *what*, *when* and *why* you eat. Write them down (try the app, iDo Notepad) to help identify bad eating habits that are so automatic you don't notice them.

BREAK THE LINK
"To compete with old habits, practice a competing behaviour repeatedly," says Dr Kessler. Instead of going straight to the fridge, go for a quick walk. And turn off the box: TV food ads increase automatic snacking impulses.

REWRITE THE SCRIPT
Change the way you talk to yourself about food, says Dr Kessler. "Instead of 'That cake looks good', remind yourself of your goals instead: 'If I don't eat that, I'll feel better about myself'," he says.

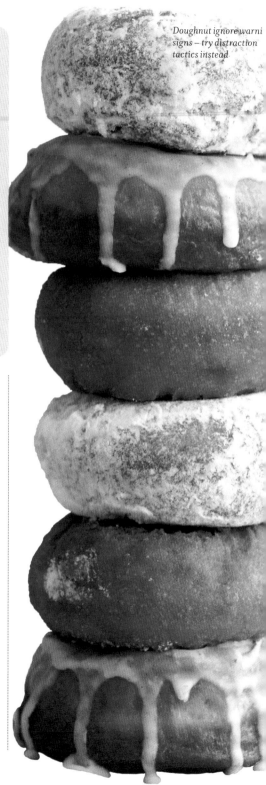

Doughnut ignore warning signs – try distraction tactics instead

Indeed, weight cycling can actually end up changing your physiology, believes Dr Brownell, who coined the term 'yo-yo dieting' in the 1980s. The more diets you've been on, the harder it becomes to lose weight. Levels of your hunger hormone ghrelin increase, and those of your fullness hormone leptin decrease, so you feel less satiated.

BORN TO REBOUND?

Dr David Kessler, author of *The End of Overeating*, and his team of researchers at the University of California at San Francisco and Yale University, looked into the biology of weight cycling. They found that the reward circuits in the brains of people Dr Kessler calls "conditioned hypereaters" were excessively activated simply by the smell of food – and stayed that way until those people finished eating whatever was on the plate in front of them. "This is a biological cause of conditioned hypereating. It's the first time we can say 'It's not your fault,'" says Dr Kessler.

Evidence shows, that this reaction is partially learned, however – and that means that through conditioning, you can rewire your brain. After all, the urge to yo-yo is not just physical; emotional triggers play a huge role too. A study at Brown University found that dieters who ate in response to emotions such as loneliness or stress – as opposed to external events, like overdoing it at happy

Losing and gaining regularly takes a huge toll on your body

hour – were more likely to regain weight.

Case in point: Darcie Schmidt lost 75lb in her late 20s, then regained a huge 120lb over two years, largely because of emotional eating, she says. In her early 30s, she stuck to a strict diet-and-exercise regime and shed 132lb. "I didn't eat a single chip for 18 months," she says. But the stress of a divorce, a move, and a return to study knocked her off track – and she ended up regaining 40lb.

Dr Oben sees women like Schmidt all the time. The problem, he believes, is that they never learned the skills needed for long-term behaviour change. "They haven't learnt how to change their mindset, and look at sensible weight maintenance and regular exercise as a lifelong thing," he says. "You need to learn how to motivate yourself and override negative thoughts."

A study of 200 people who were obese or overweight published in the *Journal of Psychosomatic Research*, supports the importance of a behaviour-change approach. Along with weight-loss techniques such as exercise and healthy eating, one group received an additional hour of acceptance-commitment therapy (ACT), where they learnt to change their behaviour; the other group just did an extra hour of low-intensity exercise.

After a year, a follow-up found that those in the therapy group had maintained their weight loss. The members of the other group had regained most or all of it. "Losing and gaining regularly takes a huge toll on your body," says

Dr Ayoob. Beyond aesthetics, such as a loss of skin elasticity, regaining weight burdens your arteries and skeletal system, and may stress the liver, which can become covered in fat.

But perhaps most startling is the dangerous and lasting effect it has on the immune system. According to the first study of the long-term impacts of yo-yo dieting, women who repeatedly lost and gained weight had poorer immune function, particularly lower counts of natural killer cells. "These cells are important for fending off infections and are also vital in fighting the early stages of cancer," says Dr Cornelia Ulrich, director of the department of preventive oncology at the National Centre for Tumour Diseases in Heidelberg, Germany. So, before you get stuck in the loop again and lose all your hard work – give these tips a go:

RETURN OF THE (BIG) MAC

Extra pounds creeping back? Shed them for good with these six strategies

1 Analyse this
Record mood and hunger levels to work out why you're eating (moodpanda.com).

2 Get snack savvy
Research published in *Diabetes Care* found that a diet rich in monounsaturated fats can help reduce belly fat. Snack on avocados, nuts and seeds.

3 Find support
Research from Birmingham University found that people who went to Weight Watchers meetings for three months lost an average of 9.7lb, compared to just 2.9lb lost by those who had one-to-one counselling at their GP's. Chat with other slimmers online at sparkpeople.com.

4 Exercise right
Cycle intensely for eight secs, then lightly for 12, for 20 mins. The University of New South Wales found women who did this lost three times more than those who cycled at a regular pace.

5 Open up
Public goals are easier to achieve, says the University of Hertfordshire. Share your goals at stickk.com.

6 Be patient
A healthy goal is to reduce your weight by around 10 per cent over six months WH

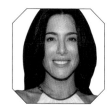

MY FLAT BELLY DIARY:

Jaime Murray

Hollywood resident, *Dexter* star and native Brit Jaime Murray is a health food lover. Let's see what flat belly ideas we can steal from across the pond

---

MONDAY

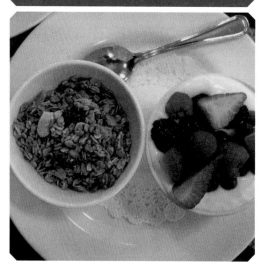

7am
Mixed berries, granola and natural yoghurt, coffee

10am
White coffee

1pm
Pret Greens and Grains No Bread salad, mixed fruit

8pm
6 oysters, sea bass with lemon quinoa salad, dark chocolate with bacon pieces

I used to have a sweet tooth, but as I've matured my tastebuds seem to have changed, even with sweet foods themselves. A while ago I would have thought that bacon chocolate was vile, but now I love a salty or savoury crunch in my dessert.

TUESDAY

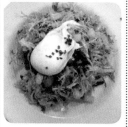

7am
Amazing Grass Chocolate Green Drink* with water and almond milk

8am
Poached egg salad with bacon and croutons, two coffees

1pm
Quinoa salad with feta and chickpeas, green pea crisps

8pm
Seabass with salad

I love to read up on nutrition. I wouldn't feel satisfied with vegetarian food, but I try to follow an alkaline diet. This chocolate-flavoured drink contains energy-upping wheatgrass.

WEDNESDAY

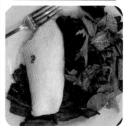

7:30am
Mixed berries and chia seeds with almond milk and natural yoghurt

1pm
Bacon omelette with salad

7:30pm
Kale salad, tuna sashimi and lentil soup

8pm
Two squares of organic dark chocolate

I'm limited for time but try to go to a spin class a minimum of four times a week. I love the anonymity and energy of classes, plus the loud music definitely helps to get me through it.

WORDS: AMELIA JEAN JONES. PHOTOGRAPHY: GETTY IMAGES. *AMAZING GRASS GREEN CHOCOLATE

THURSDAY

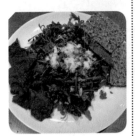

7am
Goji berries, raspberries, chia seeds in almond milk, coffee

11am
Mixed fruit

1pm
Bagel with dough removed, cream cheese and tomato, nuts

7:30pm
Salmon salad, crispbread, organic tortilla chips, glass of red wine

I never skip meals because I hate feeling hungry. Protein-rich, low-carb options (like removing the dough from my bagel) prevent me from resorting to junk food.

FRIDAY

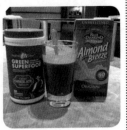

8am
Chia seeds in almond milk with yoghurt and goji berries, coffee

11am
Amazing Grass Chocolate Green Drink with water and almond milk

1pm
Tuna and egg salad on spelt flatbread

8pm
Grilled trout with lentils and rocket, glass of red wine

I go to a Bar Method class every week. It's a mixture of ballet, Pilates and yoga and strengthens the muscles with small movements. It makes everything feel tighter.

SATURDAY

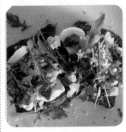

5:45am
Amazing Grass Chocolate Green Drink with water and almond milk

6:15am
Chia seeds in almond milk with yoghurt and goji berries, coffee

1pm
Egg and rocket on sprouted-grain bread, nuts

7:30pm
Salmon, potatoes, spring peas, glass of red wine

I had a long-haul flight and brought along some nutritious food. In the past, I've fallen foul of the odd cheese omelette – and felt groggy and bloated when we landed.

SUNDAY

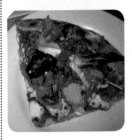

8am
Two coffees, two baked eggs, lentil and rocket salad, bread roll with butter

3pm
Mushroom soup with wholegrain crackers

8pm
Half a margherita pizza with rocket, two pan-fried sardines with broccolini

9pm
Glass of red wine

I eat out a lot at places that have simple dishes made with organic produce. When I cook, I like to experiment with new flavours – at the moment, I can't get enough of rocket.

THE EXPERT VERDICT

Our nutritional scientist Dr Christy Fergusson gives her take: "Jaime has a healthy relationship with food. She makes well-informed decisions, even when she eats out, and doesn't deprive herself.

"Just by removing the dough from her bagel, Jaime saves herself 134 calories. Her work involves a lot of travelling, so there are a few long spells of not eating. This dip in blood-sugar levels could cause an energy slump, so she should try to eat every three to four hours to prevent that.

"Fruit and nuts are great snacks to eat on the go. The combination of the carbs in the fruit along with a handful of protein-rich nuts is proven to make you feel fuller for longer, while a recovery shake within 15 minutes after a workout would give her an extra dose, too.

"Recreate Jamie's morning drink with 150ml coconut water, 100ml water, 1 serving of hemp protein powder and a tablespoon of maca. It's surprisingly tasty."

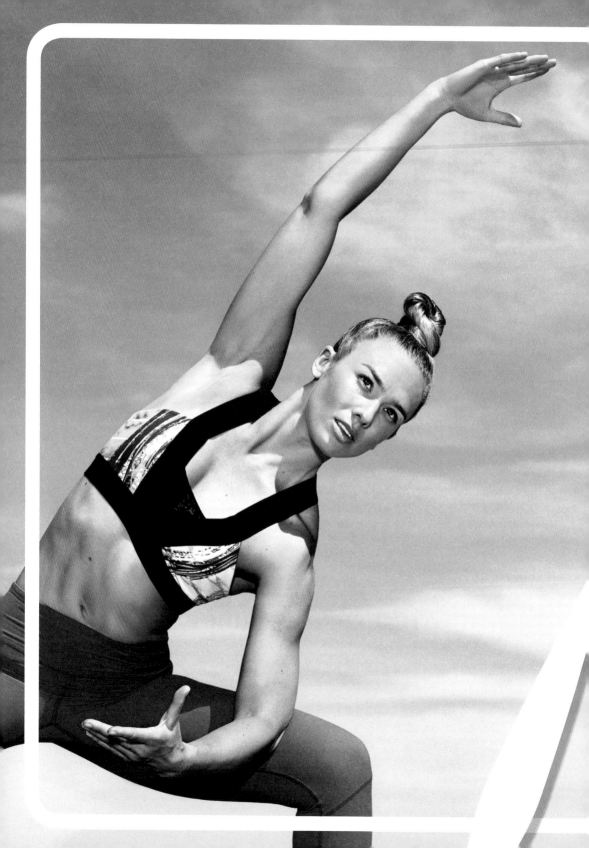

CHAPTER 5

SURE-START BREAKFASTS

Good morning! You might have woken up with a sleepy metabolism and not much fuel in the engine, but never fear – these recipes will help you kick off your flat belly day the right way. They'll fill you up with slow-burning proteins and punchy antioxidants to give you the energy you need to get you through the morning and get your body up to full fat-burning mode.

Goat's Cheese & Berry Loaf

Scones, jam and cream? So passé. This nutritious sweet-savoury breakfast will hit the spot

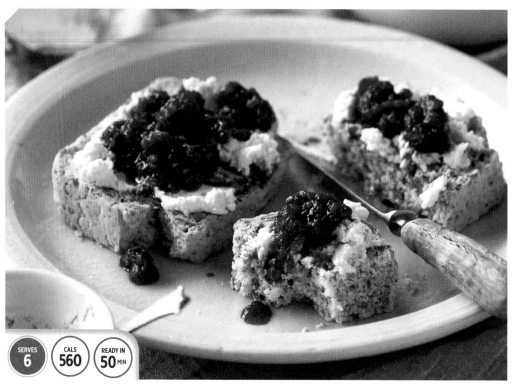

SERVES 6 · **CALS** 560 · **READY IN** 50 MIN

This tempting recipe is all about fat-blasting teamwork. The fibre-heavy coconut milk and flaxseed work together to keep you fuller for longer, the goat's cheese brings low-fat protein and the chia seeds strengthen your cell membranes to allow water and nutrients in – and toxins out. In addition to this, the raspberries are packed with antioxidants. Their vitamin D also helps to maintain your collagen stores. Now that's one hard-working toastie.

INGREDIENTS

- 350g gluten-free self-raising flour
- 30g ground flaxseed
- 20g chia seeds
- 115g mixed sunflower and pumpkin seeds
- ½ tsp sea salt
- 4 organic eggs
- 1 tsp apple cider vinegar
- 80g melted unsalted butter
- 80ml coconut milk
- 6 drops stevia liquid
- 100g fresh goat's cheese
- 2 tsp sheep's milk yoghurt
- 60g fresh raspberries

METHOD

1 It's time to dig out that loaf tin. Grease and line it (20cm x 9cm) with baking paper. Then preheat the oven to 175°C.

2 Mix the flour and all of the ground seeds in a bowl with the salt. Whisk the eggs in a separate bowl. Then stir in the vinegar, butter, coconut milk, stevia and 125ml water. Pour the wet ingredients into the bowl with the dry seed mixture and stir well.

3 Spoon the mixed ingredients into the tin and bake for 40 mins, or until a skewer inserted into the centre comes out clean. Then place it on a wire cooling rack. It will keep for a week in the fridge or two months in the freezer.

4 Mash the goat's cheese and yoghurt and spread it over two slices of the bread, toasted. Top them with a layer of slightly mashed raspberries.

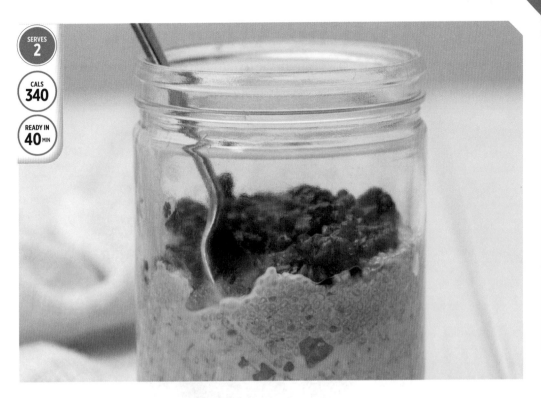

SERVES
2

CALS
340

READY IN
40 MIN

Orange Blossom & Chia Pot

Wake up, smell the coffee and make this tasty pot to fill you up for the day

Where would we be without the mighty chia seed? It's sky-high in protein, omega-3 and fibre – all essential ingredients in the fat-burning recipe. Other health benefits include stabilising blood sugar and lowering cholesterol. Plus, the seeds expand in liquid, keeping you fuller for longer. On top of this, the cinnamon and oats in this recipe both regulate insulin production, helping to keep your appetite in check until lunchtime.

INGREDIENTS
- 2 tbsp chia seeds
- 4 tbsp rice milk
- 70g porridge oats
- zest and juice of 1 orange
- 115g chopped dates
- ¼ tsp orange blossom water
- 1 cinnamon stick
- 1 punnet berries

METHOD

1 Soak the chia seeds in a bowl with the rice milk (or any other dairy-free milk alternative). In a separate bowl, combine the oats, orange zest and juice, dates, orange blossom water and cinnamon stick with 100ml warm water. Give it a good stir, then leave both bowls to sit for a minimum of 30 mins.

2 In a small glass or a jar, place a layer of berries, a layer of the orange blossom muesli, then the chia seeds, then another layer of berries of your choice on top (raspberries are a colourful option). Serve it up as a breakfast or dessert, depending on the occasion. Dig in, bliss out.

Morning-After Eggs

Don't undo your hard work. Step away from the fry-up and cook this balanced meal instead

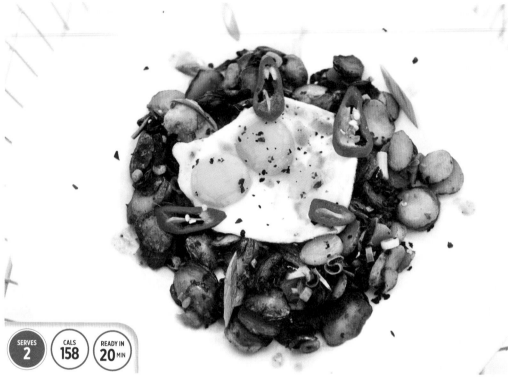

SERVES 2 | **CALS** 158 | **READY IN** 20 MIN

When you wake up after a night on the wine and find yourself reaching for your usual greasy hangover fix – give this fail-safe recovery brekkie a go instead. The eggs are full of protein to settle your stomach and stop you reaching for that bacon butty, and the chilli will kick your metabolism back into gear. Iron-rich spinach replenishes stores of potassium – a crucial electrolyte for digestive functions that are depleted when we drink.

INGREDIENTS
- 300g new potatoes
- 2 red chillis, sliced
- 2 handfuls spinach
- 4 spring onions, chopped
- 2 free-range eggs
- 1 tsp olive oil
- Knob of butter

METHOD

1. Slice the potatoes and put into a small frying pan. Cover with water, add salt and simmer until tender. Drain, wipe the pan dry and pour in the oil.

2. Fry the chilli in the pan for a minute, then tip the potatoes back in. Chuck in the butter and give the potatoes a light squish with the back of a fork.

3. Keep turning the spuds until they get golden and crispy. Then toss in the spinach and spring onions and stir until the spinach has wilted. Make a hole in the middle and crack in the eggs. Season.

4. Cook until the egg whites are set but the yolks are runny. Top with lots of chilli, then hit the sofa and enjoy.

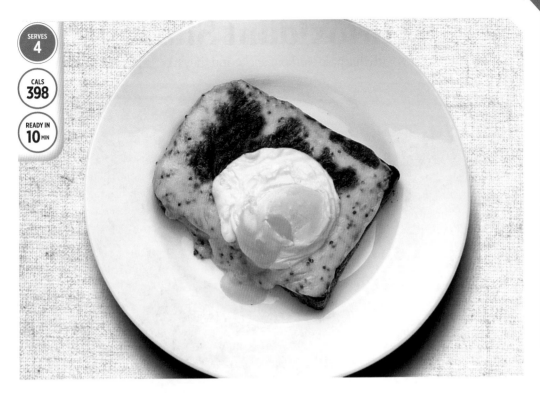

SERVES
4

CALS
398

READY IN
10 MIN

Buck Rarebit

Believe it: cheese, ale and butter, all in one meal, is nutritious and keeps hunger at bay

Hey, it's fine if last night's guests barely made a dent in your cheese board – make it a key ingredient in your brekkie instead. As well as being full of flavour, cheese packs calcium, which helps keep your appetite in check. Eggs provide vitamins A, D and E, as well as high-quality protein. You'll get a slow release of energy from the carbs in the brown bread and, along with the eggs, this will keep you full until lunch. Bye bye, biscuits.

INGREDIENTS
- 200g block of mature cheddar, or any other strong cheese
- 25g butter
- 25g plain white flour
- 2 tsp Worcestershire sauce
- 2 slugs of milk (full fat)
- 1 slug pale ale
- 4 eggs
- 1 egg yolk
- 2 large dollops of wholegrain mustard
- 4 thick slices brown bread

METHOD

1 Preheat your grill while you warm the milk and ale in a pan. Then melt the butter in a separate pan and add the flour. Cook for 2 mins, stirring slowly throughout, then whisk in the milk. Mix until smooth, then remove from the heat and beat in the cheese, egg yolk, mustard and sauce.

2 Now to poach the eggs: heat a pot of water and when it starts to boil, crack the eggs and swiftly pour them in. Cook for 4 mins, then remove them from the pot. They should feel soft and springy when a teaspoon is gently pushed against them.

3 Now, simply toast your bread, spread on the cheese and grill until golden-brown. Serve with the eggs, poached.

Antioxidant Shake

Treat your muscles with this post-workout shake and they'll burn fat all day. It's a deal

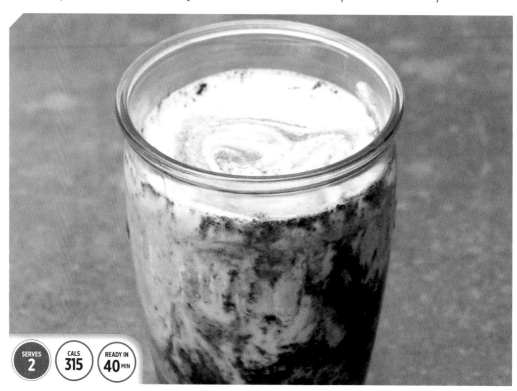

SERVES 2 | **CALS** 315 | **READY IN** 40 MIN

After a morning gym session, you'll need this antioxidant-filled milkshake in your life. Why? Because cashews are full of magnesium, an electrolyte that helps muscles to relax after hitting the gym. Plus, they are a great sources of protein for muscle recovery and, gram for gram, contain more of it than eggs. Meanwhile, baobab powder contains more energising iron than red meat. So, get blending.

INGREDIENTS
- 100g cashew nuts
- 70g frozen blueberries
- ½ tsp beetroot powder
- ½ tsp baobab powder
- 1 tsp lucuma powder

METHOD

1 To help the cashew nuts blend, soak them in 250ml of cool water for 30 mins.

2 Blend the frozen blueberries, beetroot powder and baobab powder until it forms a smooth paste. Pour it into the bottom of a glass, then give the blender a rinse. If you want to create the swirly layers like the picture, blend the blueberry mixture and the cashew milk (step 3) separately – either way will taste the same.

3 Pour the cashews and the water in which they were soaking into the blender with the lucuma powder (a natural sweetener made from the Peruvian lucuma fruit – full of B vitamins and fibre) and blend until smooth. Add water to thin it, if necessary.

4 Slowly pour this cashew 'milk' over the top of the blueberry mixture slowly to create a marbled effect. Art, darling.

BIG TABLE, BUSY KITCHEN BY ALLEGRA MCEVEDY (£25, QUERCUS)

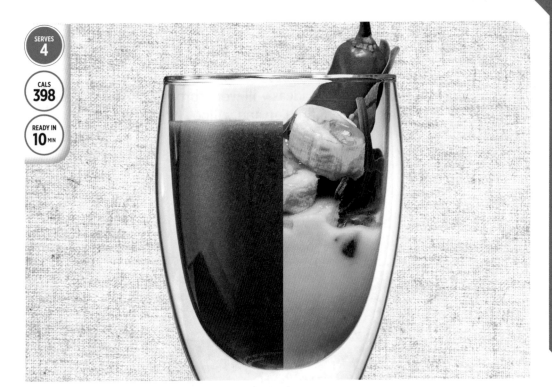

SERVES
4

CALS
398

READY IN
10 MIN

Fat-Burning Green Machine

Simply blend your way to a faster metabolism and get an ample supply of vitamins, too

This hot smoothie has flat-belly benefits all round. The potassium in the banana and chilli is great for speeding up a sluggish winter metabolism, helping to burn more fat on the go. Fructose-based honey is low-GI, so no sudden blood sugar spikes. And why heated? Well, spinach is easier to break down at this temperature, meaning the vitamins A and K, iron, manganese and folate go straight where your body needs them.

INGREDIENTS
- *1 banana*
- *125ml water*
- *125ml almond milk*
- *Handful spinach*
- *1 tsp honey*
- *⅓ tsp chilli flakes*

METHOD

1 Peel the banana and zap it in a blender along with all the other ingredients until the mixture is smooth and creamy.

2 Pour the mixture into a saucepan and heat gently until it's simmering rather than boiling.

3 Stir throughout, then pour into a mug to instantly spice up your morning.

10 Super Starts

These healthy, filling breakfast ideas will work through the day to keep your metabolism fired up and willpower intact

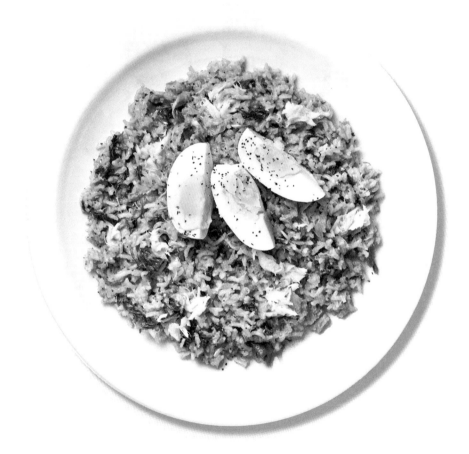

1: SLOW-BURN KEDGEREE
SERVES 1 | CALS 671 | READY IN 25 MINS

½ red onion, finely chopped • ½ tsp curry powder • 75g brown basmati rice • 1 handful baby spinach • 1 smoked mackerel fillet • 2 large hard-boiled free-range eggs

Look no further than this breakfast superhero for flat belly fuel – it's bursting with omega-3, B vitamins, slow-burn carbohydrates and metabolism-boosting spices. Begin by sautéing the onion in a little oil, until softened.

Add the curry powder and rice, and top with enough water to cover it. Simmer for 20 mins, and stir in the spinach before tearing up and adding the mackerel. Plate up, cut the eggs into wedges and place on top – then dig in.

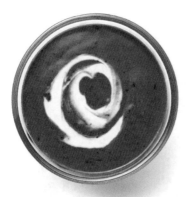

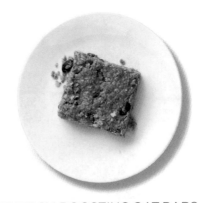

2: DE-BLOAT SEED & BERRY CRUNCH
SERVES 1 | CALS 494 | READY IN 2 MINS

150g probiotic natural yoghurt • 50g fresh blueberries • 50g fresh blackberries • 1 tbsp pumpkin seeds • 1 tbsp sunflower seeds • 30g oats

Whizz up the yoghurt and berries in a blender. Grab a fancy glass, pour in the seeds, a layer of the smoothie mix, then oats. Repeat until the glass is filled with the prettiest combination of fat-burning omega-3s and antioxidants around.

3: ENERGY-BOOSTING OAT BARS
SERVES 12 | CALS PER BAR 194 | READY IN 20 MINS

1 tbsp honey • 2 tbsp coconut oil • 2 tbsp peanut butter (no added salt or sugar) • 280g oats • 3 tbsp ground flax seeds • 1 tbsp pumpkin seeds • 2 tbsp chopped dates

Hungry by 11am? Ditch the croissant for protein-rich nuts and fat-burning seeds. Melt the honey, oil and peanut butter in a pan, then mix in the other ingredients. Press into a greased baking tin (20cm x 20cm) and bake for 10-15 mins.

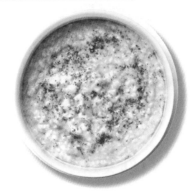

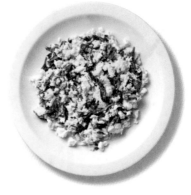

4: MAPLE & FLAX POWER PORRIDGE
SERVES 1 | CALS 551 | READY IN 10 MINS

50g oats • 250ml skimmed milk or try rice milk • 1 scoop vanilla whey protein • 1 tbsp good-quality maple syrup • 1 tbsp ground flax seeds • Pinch of cinnamon

Add the oats to a pan and cover with the milk. Turn up the stove to full heat and simmer for 5-8 mins. Take off the heat and stir in the whey protein powder and syrup. Pour into a bowl, top with the flax and cinnamon and fill up.

5: PROTEIN-PACKED SCRAMBLE
SERVES 1 | CALS 376 | READY IN 5 MINS

2 handfuls baby spinach • 2 large free-range eggs • 100g feta cheese (cubed)

Sauté the iron-rich spinach in olive oil until it has wilted. Now whisk up the eggs and add to the spinach, toss in the cubed feta, and keep stirring until the eggs are scrambled. And that's it – you're done and ready to reward your muscles.

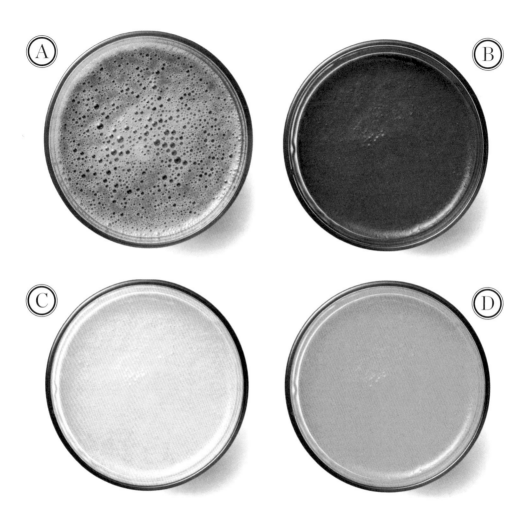

Turbo Smoothies

All these antioxidant-rich, low-calorie blends take less than two minutes to make and will sustain energy levels all day. Just pop in the blender and blitz away

6: GREEN MACHINE
SERVES 1 | CALS 251
300ml fresh pressed apple juice • 1 handful spinach • 1 handful kale • 1 banana

7: CHOCOLATE INDULGENCE
SERVES 1 | CALS 365
250ml skimmed or soy milk • 1 banana • 2 tbsp good quality pure cocoa powder • 2 tsp honey

8: PERFECTION PINA COLADA
SERVES 1 | CALS 397
Half a fresh pineapple, peeled and chopped • $^2/_3$ cans light coconut milk • 1 scoop vanilla whey protein

9: MARVELLOUS MANGO LASSI
SERVES 1 | CALS 302
1 fresh mango, peeled and chopped • 200g natural probiotic yogurt

10: TRIPLE-THREAT FRITTATA
SERVES 1 | CALS 589 | READY IN 15 MINS

2 large free-range eggs
• ½ cooked beetroot, cut into small chunks • 1 small smoked mackerel fillet
• 45g goat's cheese

Could your post-gym muscles do better than this omega-3 rich, three-protein hit? They'll repay you by burning fat, you know. Whisk the eggs in a bowl with a little salt and pepper. Add the beetroot to a frying pan, along with a little olive oil. Sauté for 1 min, pour on the whisked eggs, flake in the mackerel fillet right away (no skin please), and crumble in the goat's cheese. Cook for about 3 mins on the stove, before placing the pan under a hot grill to cook the top. This should take about 3-4 mins, or until it begins to firm up.

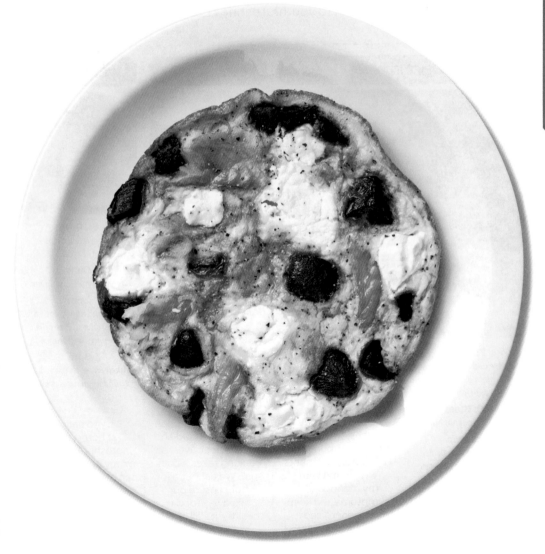

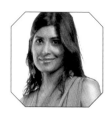

MY FLAT BELLY DIARY:

Ruby Hammer

Has Ruby Hammer, make-up artist and co-founder of Ruby & Millie cosmetics, found the secret to youthful eating? Let's investigate

MONDAY

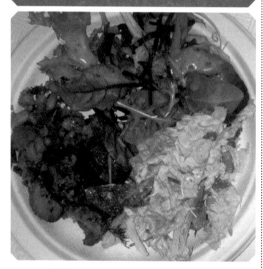

7:30am
Orange and lime juice with Udo's Choice oil, crumpet and jam, tea with milk and sugar

10:30am
Toast with peanut butter

2:30pm
Green salad with beans, ratatouille and potatoes

8:30pm
Chicken soup with avocado

I regularly take Udo's Choice Ultimate Oil Blend and black cohosh, which is a herb that can reduce hot flushes, which I get from my acupuncturist. I rely on supplements to help me with my menopausal symptoms and keep me energised through the day.

TUESDAY

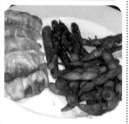

7am
Water, herbal tea

8:30am
Boiled egg, half a croissant, tea with milk and sugar

2pm
Udon noodles with sea bream

4:30pm
A protein ball

8pm
Edamame, asparagus and chicken gyoza

I'm not the best chef, plus my husband and I have hectic lives, so cooking takes a back seat. We eat out a lot, but I ensure our takeaway food is healthy. It's all about convenience.

WEDNESDAY

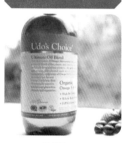

8:30am
Orange and lime juice, Udo's oil

9am
Tea with milk and sugar

2pm
Falafel and hummus wrap, crisps, olives, feta-stuffed peppers and grapes

8pm
Takeaway of chapati, dahl and lamb rogan josh

I try to eat clean at home, but at photoshoots I'm at the mercy of caterers. This can mean nibbling side dishes, especially if the main meal is pork-based – I'm Muslim so I don't eat it.

AS TOLD TO: AMELIA JEAN JONES. PHOTOGRAPHY: GETTY IMAGES

THURSDAY	FRIDAY	SATURDAY	SUNDAY

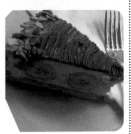 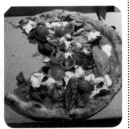 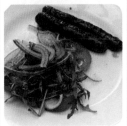 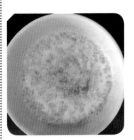

THURSDAY

8am
Porridge with maple syrup and tea with milk and sugar

11am
A kiwi, green tea

2pm
Grilled chicken, sweet potatoes, banoffee pie

5pm
Bombay mix

9pm
Spaghetti pomodoro

I'm lucky to have good skin, but staying youthful isn't all about make-up. I try to curb my sweet tooth as sugar causes wrinkles, but I sometimes fail and have banoffee pie!

FRIDAY

8:30am
Tea with milk and sugar

2pm
Chilli con carne with wild rice and carrot salad

4:30pm
Herbal tea

8pm
Three slices of basil, mozzarella, rocket and red pepper pizza

8:30pm
Green tea

I don't think it's healthy to deny yourself anything – you sit there thinking and that leads to binge eating. If I want pizza, I just eat a small amount of my favourite kind.

SATURDAY

9am
Cottage cheese and pineapple on Ryvita, tea with milk and sugar

1:30pm
Sausages with avocado and rocket, orange and lime juice

7pm
Edamame with squid, black cod, rice, asparagus

8pm
2 lychee martinis

My father was a doctor and he always told me not to drink liquid when you eat because it dilutes your digestive juices. I always have a drink before or after a meal, never during.

SUNDAY

9am
Porridge with maple syrup, tea with milk and sugar

2pm
Chilli con carne with long grain and wild rice, carrot salad and sweet potatoes

4pm
A packet of sweet popcorn

9pm
Shepherd's pie

Since my mum died two years ago, I've found it hard to motivate myself to go to the gym. Instead, I like to go for brisk, two-hour walks at weekends.

THE EXPERT VERDICT

Nutritionist Dr Christy Fergusson gives her feedback: "Ruby's main problem is her breakfasts, which are fairly high in sugar and low in good-quality protein.

"Some mornings she only has tea with milk and sugar, or amps up her slow-energy-releasing oats with sugary maple syrup. Stimulants like caffeine and sugar cause hot flushes (not ideal if, like Ruby, you're experiencing menopausal symptoms), while excess sugar gets dumped on the skin and speeds up the ageing process.

"A green juice or smoothie would be a better start to her day. Throwing in an avocado would add protein and good-quality fats to balance her hormones and skin, too.

"Udo's Choice oil is a great addition, though. It's a perfect balance of omegas 3, 6 and 9. She's also right about drinking water with meals, but sipping apple cider vinegar in a little water with food aids digestion. Just don't pair it with oily chips!"

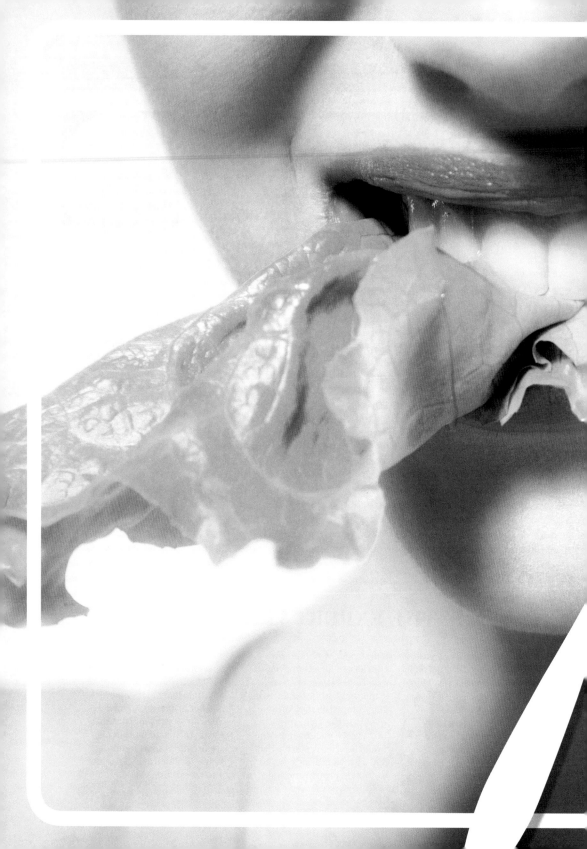

CHAPTER 6

POWER LUNCHES

Commute, office, workout... it's easier to run out for a sandwich, surely? Think again: as well as taking pounds from your purse a fast-burning baguette will be adding them to your weight, too. We've come up with these delicious recipes to fuel your work and exercise and fend off afternoon cookie cravings. Make in minutes, enjoy through your lunch hour – lose weight for good.

Moroccan Lamb Soup

Hosting a lunch? Impress all with your international, calorie-conscious cooking skills

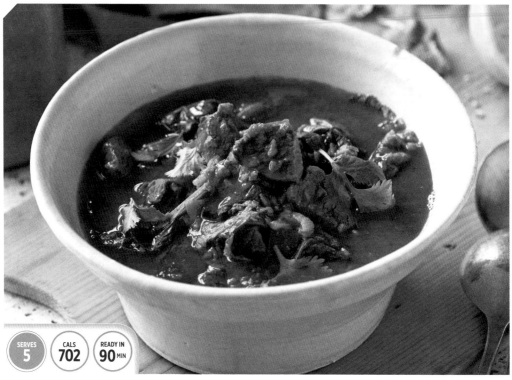

SERVES 5

CALS 702

READY IN 90 MIN

Look at the back of your kitchen cupboard: the humble lentil is your flat belly ally. It provides a slow release of energy that, along with the lamb's protein, will make you feel full for longer – and less prone to nibbling before dinner. While there's no better way of beating a post-meal belly bloat than ginger, it also contains the antioxidant gingerol, which tones up your skin and prevents ageing. That's what we call multitasking.

INGREDIENTS

- 2 tbsp extra-virgin olive oil
- 1kg diced lamb (shoulder or leg), fat trimmed off
- 1 onion, thinly sliced
- 1 tbsp ground turmeric
- 1 tbsp ground ginger
- 1 tbsp ground cinnamon
- 1 tbsp harissa
- 215g lentils
- 2 litres chicken stock
- 1 large tomato, diced
- Juice of 1 lemon
- 1 bunch baby spinach
- 1 bunch coriander, to serve

METHOD

1 Heat 1 tbsp of the olive oil in a pan, then add the lamb and sear for 5 mins. Remove from the heat and set aside.

2 Add the remaining oil to a large saucepan over a high heat. Add the onion and cook for 3 mins, stirring, until it has caramelised. Turn the heat down to medium and then stir in the turmeric, ginger and cinnamon. Cook for another 3 mins.

3 Add the lamb to the pan and mix well. Stir in the harissa and lentils, then the chicken stock. Reduce the heat and simmer, covered, for 1 hour.

4 Add the tomato, lemon juice and spinach and simmer for 5 mins. Then turn off the heat and serve topped with the coriander.

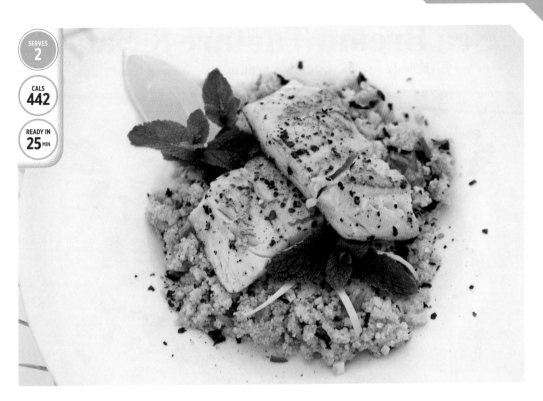

SERVES
2

CALS
442

READY IN
25 MIN

Haddock & Cauli Couscous

No illusions here; this is all good stuff that will keep you, well, stuffed

Pick a carb, any carb – we guarantee that you won't miss the usual fast-burn couscous that we've swapped for low-GI cauliflower. It won't just keep you fuller for longer; glucosinolates help aid detoxification and, with the lemon, it "cleanses the digestive system," says nutritionist Vicki Edgson. The magic doesn't stop there; the haddock is teeming with omega-3, essential for post-gym muscle recovery. And for our next trick...

INGREDIENTS
- 2 lemons
- 180g haddock
- 35ml olive oil
- 1 cauliflower
- ½ tsp turmeric
- ¼ bunch mint
- 100g Greek yoghurt
- Salt and pepper
- 25g tahini
- ½ clove garlic, minced

METHOD

1 Squeeze the juice of half a lemon over the fish. Place it skin-side down on a lightly oiled tray under a grill for 4 mins. Flip and grill for a further minute or until the skin is crispy.

2 Break up the cauliflower and toss with the turmeric and 25ml oil. Season and roast at 180°C until tender.

3 Cool, then blitz in a processor until it resembles couscous. Chop the mint and add to the cauliflower with the zest of one lemon.

4 To make the tahini cream, mix the yoghurt, tahini, juice of half a lemon, garlic, 10ml oil, 20ml water and season. Whisk until thick.

5 Spoon cauliflower on two plates, place the fish on top and drizzle over cream.

Sea Bream Tartare & Salad

The tasty-ass, fancy-pants way to fill up and slim your tummy

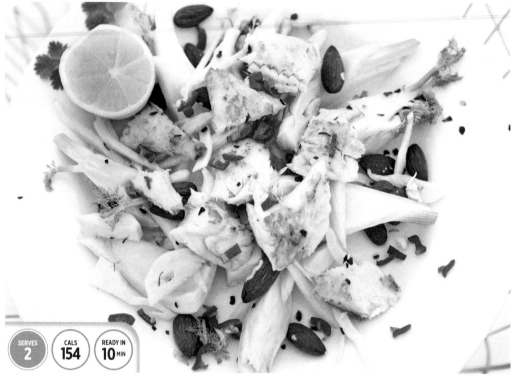

SERVES 2 | **CALS** 154 | **READY IN** 10 MIN

Is there a prettier way of fending off the afternoon munchies? We don't think so. There's some serious muscle hiding behind this princess of a dish: the low-fat protein of the sea bream and the fat-fighting almonds will keep your appetite at bay all afternoon. Meanwhile, the fennel's high doses of antioxidants will help streamline your digestion, while the chilli revs your metabolism for hours afterwards. Perfection.

INGREDIENTS

- 1 medium fennel, finely sliced
- 3 tsp lemon juice
- 20ml extra-virgin olive oil
- 10 salted almonds
- Salt and pepper
- 2 sea bream fillets
- 1 tsp red chilli, finely chopped
- 2 tbsp Greek yoghurt

METHOD

1 This one is really simple. Mix the fennel, 1 tsp of the lemon juice, the olive oil and the almonds in a bowl, then season with salt and pepper and set aside. No nibbling now.

2 Remove the skin and any small bones from the sea bream (get your tweezers out – just kidding), then cut it into cubes.

3 Season the bream with the chilli, Greek yoghurt, salt and pepper and remaining lemon juice and serve immediately with the fennel and almond mix.

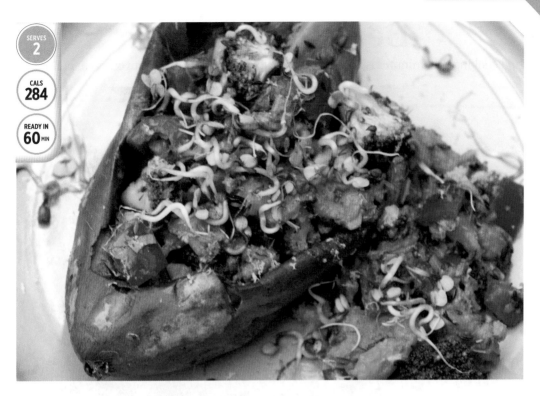

SERVES
2

CALS
284

READY IN
60 MIN

Stuffed Sweet Potato

Standard spuds got upgraded: this option is more nutritious, lower in fat and guilt-free

Sweet potatoes can do no wrong in the flat belly universe; pack this bad boy for your lunch and you won't find yourself reaching for the cookie jar. High-fibre and low calorie, it's quicker to list the metabolism-boosting vitamins it *doesn't* contain, and its high iron content will make sure any protein – in this case, feta – is effectively processed and sent straight to your muscles. Gym heaven.

INGREDIENTS

- 2 medium-size sweet potatoes
- 2 tbsp melted coconut oil
- 1 clove garlic, grated
- ¼ tsp caraway seeds
- ¼ cup water
- 60g broccoli florets, chopped
- 1 red pepper, diced
- 20g chopped parsley
- Juice and zest of 1 lemon
- 7g fresh dill, chopped
- Salt
- 20g feta

METHOD

1 Preheat the oven to 175°C, cover the sweet potato in 1 tbsp coconut oil and a sprinkle of salt, then bake on a tray for 50 mins.

2 Remove it from the oven and cut a slit lengthways down the centre. Gently scoop the flesh into a bowl. (Beware, it's hot!)

3 In a frying pan, heat the rest of the coconut oil with the garlic and caraway seeds. Cook for 1 min, then add half of the water, plus all the broccoli, pepper and parsley. Cook for a further 2 mins.

4 Add the lemon juice and the sweet potato flesh to the pan, then cook for 2 mins. Stir in the rest of the water, lemon zest and dill. Don't forget to season with salt.

5 Stuff the mixture into the sweet potato skins and serve with a sprinkle of sprouts or herbs and feta cheese to garnish.

Beetroot Tartare

Sod cooking – 15 minutes is all you need to pack in protein and boost your gym endurance

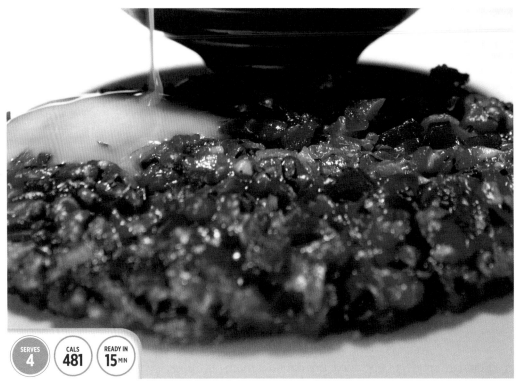

SERVES 4   **CALS** 481   **READY IN** 15 MIN

It's a raw classic, packed with protein. But if you're apprehensive about uncooked beef, think about the gym benefits and then give it a try. This variation of the classic dish substitutes half of the steak for beetroot – and for good reason. A study by the University of Exeter showed juiced beets improve exercise endurance by 16 per cent. This recipe also sneaks in energising, iron-packed capers and vitamin C-rich parsley. Go on, try it.

INGREDIENTS
- 400g cooked beetroot
- 160g beef fillet
- 40g shallots, peeled and chopped
- 40g capers
- 40g gherkins, chopped
- 1 tbsp honey
- 1 tbsp white wine vinegar
- 1 bunch parsley, chopped
- 4 egg yolks
- 4 slices wholemeal bread

METHOD

1 Ready for your Michelin moment? Drain the beetroot and cut it into tiny cubes. (And keep white clothes out of sight!)

2 Next, chop the beef fillet into cubes of the same size and mix with the beets. Fold in the shallots, capers and gherkins. Then add the honey, vinegar and parsley, stirring gently. Season to taste.

3 Gently fold in the egg yolks, cover with cling film (making sure the film touches the surface of the mix) and refrigerate for an hour. Put your serving plates in the fridge.

4 Divide the tartare onto the four cold plates, shaping them to create a uniform, round circle. If you want to spice it up, add a few drops of Tabasco. Serve with triangles of wholemeal toast if you need a carb hit.

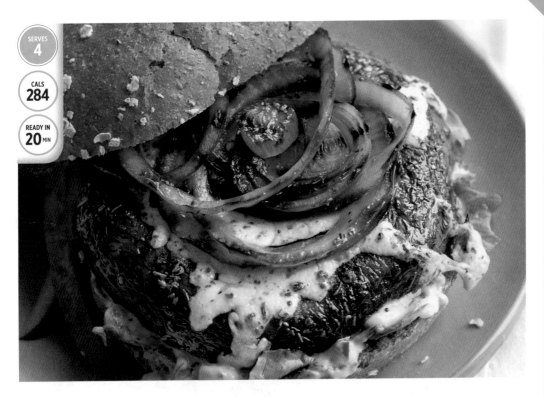

SERVES
4

CALS
284

READY IN
20 MIN

Veggie Burger with Mayo

Many burgers – beef or veg – are laced with hidden fat and salt. But this one's a tasty, safe bet

Veggie burgers may seem safe for non-meat eaters and calorie counters alike. But the truth is, they offer little or no improvement from the overload of calories, fat and salt in beef burgers. The smart alternative? A meaty Portobello mushroom, rubbed in olive oil and balsamic, topped with a crown of melted mozzarella. Even if you're a beef buff, we think you'll like this one. There's plenty of flavour to get your teeth into.

INGREDIENTS

- 2 tbsp mayonnaise
- Juice of ½ lemon
- ½ jar roasted red peppers
- 1 clove garlic, crushed
- 4 large Portobello mushrooms, stems removed
- 1 tbsp olive oil
- 1 tbsp balsamic vinegar
- 1 tsp dried Italian seasoning
- Handful grated mozzarella
- 1 red onion, sliced into rings
- 4 wholemeal buns
- A few handfuls of lettuce, rocket or any green salad leaves

METHOD

1 Combine the mayonnaise, lemon juice, red peppers and garlic. If you want a uniformly red mayonnaise, purée the lot for a few seconds in a food processor.

2 Heat a griddle pan (or a frying pan if you don't have one). Rub the mushrooms with the olive oil, vinegar, Italian seasoning, salt and pepper. Place the mushrooms in the pan and top them with the mozzarella. Cook for 2 to 3 mins, until the cheese is melted and the mushrooms are fully cooked.

3 While the mushrooms are cooking, fry the onions in another pan until brown. Slice and toast the buns, either under the grill for 2 mins or in a toaster.

4 Place each mushroom in a bun and top with greens, fried onions and the red pepper mayonnaise.

Risi e Bisi

Super hungry? Tuck into this hearty, filling Italian rice dish. *Delizioso*

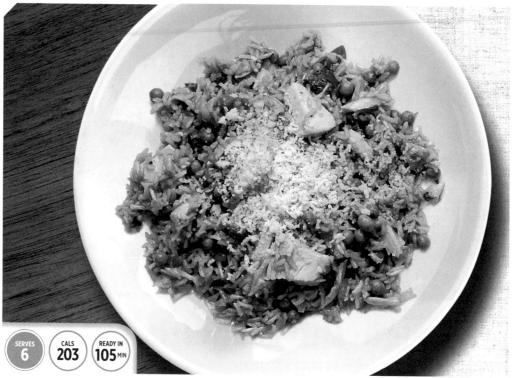

SERVES **6** CALS **203** READY IN **105** MIN

The secret to steering clear of the snack cupboard? Eat healthy, filling meals every three to four hours. This dish has the perfect mix of brown, low-GI carbs (such as brown rice) and lean protein (like turkey) to keep you going until dinner. It's flavoured with iron and vitamin C-packed herbs, bacon – which brings B vitamins and omega-3 – and calcium-filled Parmesan. And you can put your feet up while it slow-cooks on the hob.

INGREDIENTS

- 3 small onions (1 whole, 2 chopped)
- 1 carrot
- 1 celery stick
- 2 rosemary sprigs
- 2 bay leaves
- 1 large bunch of parsley
- 1 large bunch thyme
- 120g cooked turkey
- 25g butter
- 1 tsp olive oil
- 2 rashers of bacon
- 200g brown basmati rice
- 75g peas (frozen or fresh)
- 2 tsp Parmesan (optional)

METHOD

1 Start by putting the whole onion, carrot, celery and herbs into a large saucepan. Cover with two litres of water, bring to the boil and simmer for 45 mins.

2 Add the turkey and then leave the pot to simmer for another 15 mins. Then strain the stock into another saucepan, set aside the turkey and discard the rest.

3 Next, heat the butter and olive oil in a deep frying pan before sweating the sliced onions and bacon. Add the rice and gradually stir in about 500ml of the stock. Cook for 45 mins, then turn off the heat.

4 Stir in the peas, leave for 5 mins and add the turkey, parsley (and Parmesan if you're feeling like treating yourself).

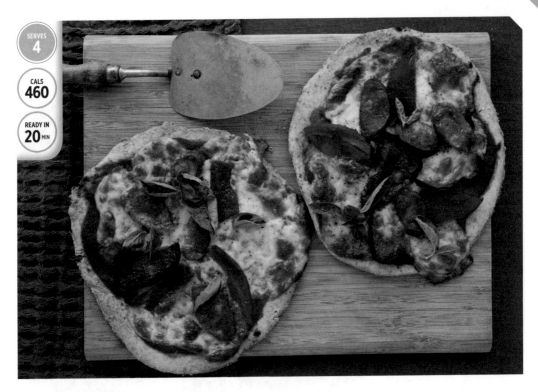

SERVES
4

CALS
460

READY IN
20 MIN

Red Pepper & Chorizo Pizza

Go DIY on naughty food. This recipe gives a classic dish a healthy twist

We know you're craving a treat, but step away from the takeaway pizza menu and head to the kitchen for a home-made deal. The brown base will give you a sustained release of energy, rather than the sudden boom and bust you get from white carbs. The red peppers contain 300 per cent (and no, that's not a typo) of your daily metabolism-supporting vitamin C requirements.

INGREDIENTS

- 1 onion, sliced
- 1 punnet cherry tomatoes
- 2 cloves garlic, crushed
- 1 red pepper, seeded and quartered
- 4 tbsp olive oil
- 1 tsp sugar
- 2 wholegrain pizza bases
- 300g mozzarella, sliced
- 2 red peppers, seeded and quartered
- 2 chorizo sausages, sliced diagonally
- Handful of fresh basil

METHOD

1 First, preheat your oven to 220°C. Now place the onion, tomatoes, garlic, pepper, olive oil and sugar in a large roasting pan and roast for 30 mins.

2 Remove from the oven and purée with a food processor or hand-held blender until smooth. Now just leave your mix to cool before blobbing 3 tbsp on top of each pizza base, spreading evenly. Keep the rest in the fridge for another meal.

3 Now chuck on the cheese, red peppers and that juicy chorizo, then pop your pizzas in the oven for 15 to 20 mins or until mouth-wateringly golden brown.

4 Throw on the basil leaves while it's still hot, then get stuck in. Sharing is optional.

Sprout & Almond Medley

This guilt-free dish boasts a fruity, nutty flavour, as well as a long list of nutrients

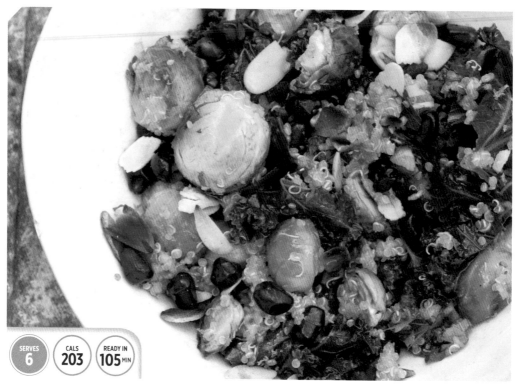

SERVES 6 · **CALS** 203 · **READY IN** 105 MIN

Kale isn't just one of the best sources of iodine, iron, calcium and potassium – it also revs up your digestion with its high fibre content. Combine that with sprouts, which are filled with glucosinolates (amazing little things that help your liver eliminate toxins) and you have a detox-on-a-plate that doesn't involve liquid meals. And it's not all green leaves – the dressing will tickle your tongue while the quinoa and almonds fill your tum.

INGREDIENTS
- 250g Brussels sprouts
- 1 clove garlic, finely chopped
- 100g quinoa
- 100g kale, chopped at 8cm intervals
- 1 tbsp olive oil
- 1 tsp rice vinegar
- 3g fresh ginger, grated
- Zest of 1 orange
- 1 tsp pomegranate molasses
- 10g chopped fresh parsley
- 30g flaked almonds
- ½ pomegranate

METHOD

1 Preheat the oven to 175°C, then chop off the sprouts' bases and cut them in half. Put them into a baking tray with the garlic and a pinch of salt. Bake for 25 mins.

2 Cook the quinoa according to the instructions on the packet and drain. Now set a stopwatch and boil kale in salted water for 30 to 40 seconds. Drain well.

4 In a bowl, mix the almonds, sprouts, quinoa, kale, vinegar, ginger, orange zest, pomegranate molasses and parsley.

5 Brown the almonds in a pan for 1 min over a low heat. Now, hold half each pomegranate at a time, sliced side facing down, and bang the top with the back of a wooden spoon to dislodge the seeds. Serve the salad hot or cold and garnish with the pomegranate seeds and almonds.

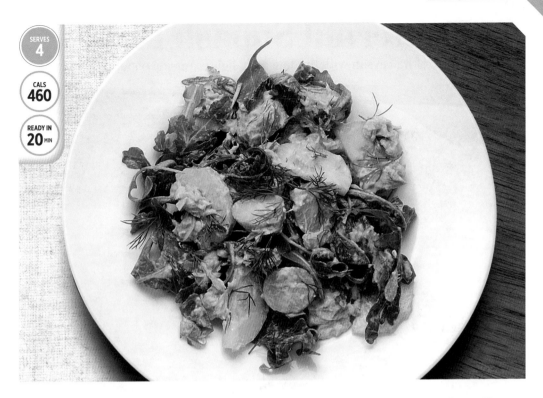

Fat-Torching Salmon Salad

A fresh-fish dish with a bit of a kick. Tuck into this salad for maximum body-benefits

Omega-3-loaded salmon is the fish that keeps on giving – or in the case of your waistline, helps take away. This recipe combines a balance of protein from the fish and yoghurt, and carbs from the potatoes to help you stay fuller for longer. Meanwhile, the chilli from the Tabasco and the wasabi and horseradish give your taste buds a kick while firing up your metabolism. It's time to feel the burn.

INGREDIENTS

- 75g salmon, baked or poached
- 1 tsp grated horseradish
- 250g natural low-fat yoghurt
- Juice of 1 lemon
- Tabasco (to taste)
- 1 splash of white wine vinegar
- Wasabi paste (to taste)
- 1 medium cucumber, peeled and sliced
- Fresh dill
- 100g potatoes, boiled
- Wild rocket

METHOD

1 Start by flaking the salmon into a bowl. Now in another bowl mix the horseradish, yoghurt, lemon juice and a couple of drops of tabasco to make your horseradish sauce.

2 Grab a jug, pour in the vinegar and blend in a small squeeze of wasabi (be careful not to overdo it). Next, pop in the chopped-up cucumber and dill with a pinch of salt. Then stir the horseradish sauce in with the sliced potatoes and add the cucumber and wasabi mix.

3 Finally, add the salmon with rocket, more dill and a squeeze of lemon. Now all that's left is to plate up and tuck in.

Butternut Squash Pizza

Enjoy a taste of Italian sun with this low-guilt, lighter version of our old favourite

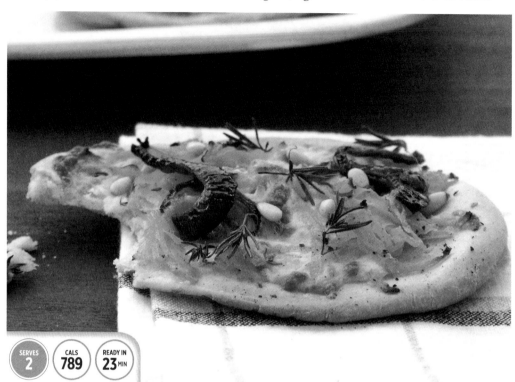

SERVES **2** · CALS **789** · READY IN **23** MIN

The pine nuts on this pizza contain pinolenic acid – an effective appetite suppressant. Useful when your pizza tastes this good. Recent research has shown that squash is packed full of antioxidants, is high in fibre and helps with blood sugar regulation.

INGREDIENTS

- *1 small red onion, cut into quarters*
- *1 tsp olive oil*
- *2 prepared pizza bases*
- *1 small butternut squash, peeled and grated*
- *2 tbsp feta, roughly crumbled*
- *Pine nuts*
- *Sprig of fresh rosemary*

METHOD

1 Go on then, fire her up to 220°C. Pop your onion in a pan with olive oil, cover with a lid and cook for 5 mins or until soft.

2 Unleash your inner artist to decorate each base with your grated butternut, feta, pine nuts and onion.

3 Rip up the fresh rosemary and sprinkle it evenly over your pizzas, then bake for 15 to 20 mins or until as golden as Ryan Gosling's chest (yep, it's just as tasty too).

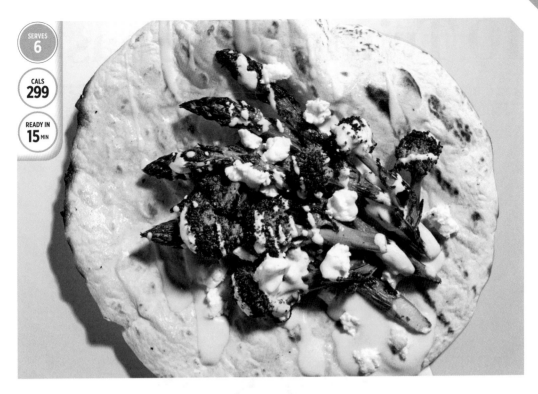

SERVES
6

CALS
299

READY IN
15 MIN

Veg Wrap with Yoghurt

Go green this lunchtime with this speedy dish, as tasty as it is trimming

Vegetarians need not get a raw deal when it comes to protein – as this Argentine recipe proves. Goat's cheese does the muscle-fuelling trick here, with up to a third less fat than the bovine kind. And there's no flavour lost even though the fat's been slashed; system-cleansing asparagus and broccoli put in double duty on that front, while the rapeseed oil and yoghurt in the tangy sauce cuts the fat content to half that of mayo. Yum.

INGREDIENTS

- 18 asparagus spears
- 2 tbsp extra-virgin olive oil
- 1 tsp chilli flakes
- 300g purple sprouting broccoli, blanched
- 3 tbsp French mustard
- 6 wholemeal tortilla wraps
- 300g goat's cheese
- 2 tbsp rapeseed oil
- 1 tbsp cider vinegar
- 120ml plain, non-fat Greek yoghurt
- 2 tsp honey

METHOD

1 First, snap off the tough ends of the asparagus and put the good bits in a large bowl with 1 tbsp oil, sea salt, pepper and the chilli flakes. Set aside for 1 hour.

2 Do exactly the same thing with the blanched broccoli, only put the crispy stems in a bowl with the rest of the oil, the seasoning and half the mustard.

3 Grill the asparagus and broccoli for 5-10 mins, until nicely charred. Towards the end, grill your tortilla wraps on both sides.

4 In a small bowl, whisk the rapeseed oil and vinegar together, then mix the rest of the mustard, yoghurt and honey to make your yoghurt sauce.

5 To finish, put a spoonful of yoghurt sauce on each wrap, and add the asparagus, broccoli and goat's cheese.

10 Trimming Toasts

You don't have to banish bread for a flat belly – use your loaf and choose low-GI sourdough. *MasterChef: The Professionals* winner Keri Moss, shows you how

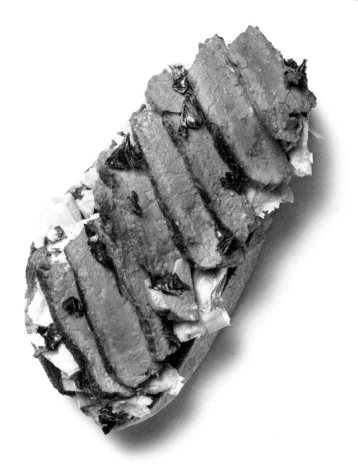

1: DETOX STEAK SARNIE

SERVES 1 | CALS 357 | READY IN 6 MINS

100g steak • Olive oil • 1 clove garlic, crushed • 80g tinned artichokes • 20g fresh grated Parmesan • 2 sprigs flat-leaf parsley, chopped

Heat a grill pan. Season the steaks. Grill for 3 mins a side and rest. Brush both sides of the bread with olive oil and garlic and then griddle both sides. Chop the artichokes and mix with the Parmesan and half the parsley. Spread the artichoke mix on the toast. Slice the steaks and put on top with the other half of the parsley. Now here's a toast boast for you: "Artichoke leaf improves the liver's eliminative function," says Amelia Hirota, herbalist clinician at the Center of Balance. Detox away.

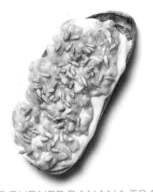

2: FAT-BURNER BANANA TOAST
SERVES 1 | CALS 207 | READY IN 5 MINS

Sprinkling of sunflower seeds • 20g low-fat soft cheese • 5g runny honey • ½ large banana, roughly mashed

Put down the cupcake and whisk up this sweet treat instead. Preheat the oven to 180°C and pop the sourdough in the toaster. Bake the sunflower seeds for 4-5 mins until golden. Mix the cheese with the honey and banana and spread on the toast, then scatter on the seeds.

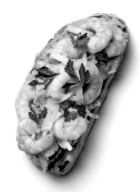

3: TONE-UP WASABI TOAST
SERVES 1 | CALS 284 | READY IN 5 MINS

Olive oil • 1 tsp wasabi paste • Juice of ½ lime • ½ tsp honey • ½ large avocado • Salt • Black pepper • 120g cooked prawns • ½ head of chicory • Sprig of parsley

A slice of metabolism-firing zinginess. Peel avocado, crush in a bowl and season, then whisk olive oil, wasabi, lime juice and honey together and mix in. Put prawns in a bowl and mix with dressing and shredded chicory. Spread avocado on the toast and top with prawns and parsley.

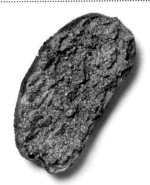

4: FAT-BUSTING PESTO PIECE
SERVES 1 | CALS 179 | READY IN 3 MINS

125g rocket • 2 cloves garlic • 50g pine nuts • 50g fresh grated Parmesan • 1 lemon, juiced • Pinch salt • Ground black pepper • 80ml olive oil

The flat belly heroes in this recipe are pine nuts, which contain hunger-busting pinolenic acid. Blend everything except the oil in a food processor until smooth. Keep it running, then slowly add the oil until you have a paste – then simply spread on toast. Presto!

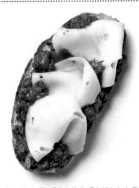

5: SLIM-DOWN CHILLI SLICE
SERVES 1 | CALS 234 | READY IN 60 MINS

4 cloves garlic • 4 red chillies • 12g fresh ginger • 30ml fish sauce • 500g tomatoes • 300g caster sugar • 100ml red wine vinegar • 1 slice Swiss cheese

Ginger and chilli love ganging up on fat – the big bullies. Whizz garlic, chillies, ginger and fish sauce in a blender, add tomatoes and pulse. Pour into a pan, add sugar and vinegar and boil. Reduce to a simmer and cook for 45 mins. Cool before serving on toast, topped with cheese.

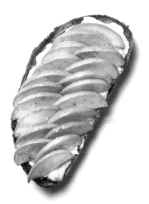

6: FAT-BURNING APPLE SLICE
SERVES 1 | CALS 148 | READY IN 3 MINS

30g light cream cheese · ½ apple, quartered · Pinch ground cinnamon · 10g agave syrup

Lightly toast a slice of sourdough, then spread the cream cheese on top and place onto a baking tray. Slice apple quarters and arrange on top of the cream cheese. Sprinkle cinnamon over the apple and drizzle with agave syrup. Place under a grill and cook till golden.

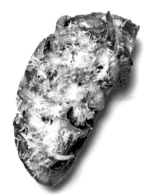

7: CLEAR-SKIN MUSHROOM CANAPÉ
SERVES 1 | CALS 480 | READY IN 20 MINS

25g butter · 1 clove garlic, chopped · 180g mushrooms, sliced · Pinch salt · A little black pepper · 1 egg · 15ml crème fraîche · 8g fresh grated Parmesan

Heat oven to 175°C. Melt a little butter in a pan, add the garlic and fry the mushrooms for 5 mins. Season and cool. Toast the bread. Mix egg with the crème fraîche and add the cooled mushrooms. Pile generously onto the toast and sprinkle with Parmesan. Bake for 12 mins.

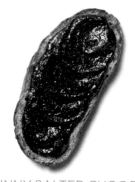

8: SKINNY SALTED CHOC BREAD
SERVES 1 | CALS 183 | READY IN 15 MINS

100g skinned whole hazelnuts · 250g quality milk chocolate, melted · 1 tbsp demerara sugar · 1 tbsp grapeseed oil · Small pinch Maldon sea salt

Roast hazelnuts for 10 mins. Whizz them into a paste in a processor with the chocolate, sugar and salt. Slowly drizzle in the grapeseed oil. Grill your toast and put the mix in the fridge to firm up before spreading. Or grab a spoon and tuck in. We know what we'd do.

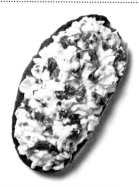

9: POST-GYM EGGS FLORENTINE
SERVES 1 | CALS 452 | READY IN 5 MINS

½ red chilli, chopped with seeds taken out · Knob of butter · 2 eggs · 30ml single cream · Black pepper · 50g baby spinach · Pinch salt · 10g fresh grated Parmesan

Perfect R&R for worked-out muscles. Fry chilli in the butter until tender. Break eggs into a bowl and mix in cream and pepper to taste. Pour into the chilli pan and stir. Add spinach and salt. Cook until the spinach has wilted and eggs are soft. Serve on the toast, topped with Parmesan.

10: FLAT-BELLY FRENCH TOAST
SERVES 1 | CALORIES 297 | READY IN 30 MINS

5g plain flour • Pinch cinnamon • Pinch brown sugar • Salt • 20ml semi-skimmed milk • 1 egg • ½ tsp vanilla extract • 2 plums • 10g caster sugar • 30g non-fat Greek yoghurt

This one may take a little longer than some of the others, but it's *so* worth it. Put the flour, cinnamon, sugar and salt in a bowl. Beat the milk, egg and vanilla in another. Whisk the milk mix into the dry mix until smooth. Chop the plums and simmer in a pan with the sugar till tender. Soak the bread in the batter and fry until lightly golden on each side. Serve with yoghurt and warm compote. Flavonoids in the plums and probiotics in yoghurt help prevent bloating. Yum!

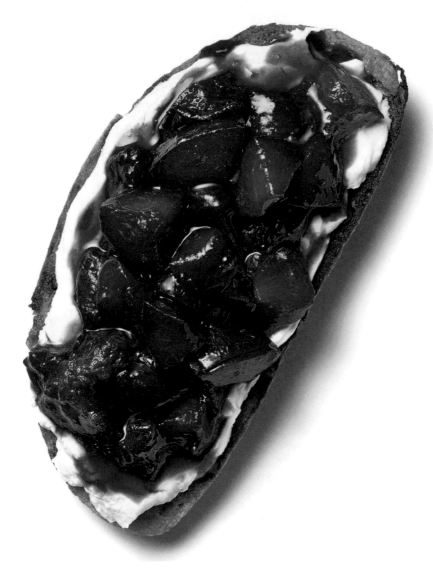

10 Clever Quinoas

Swap the carbs in your lunch for this smartypants supergrain, and its hefty
protein content will take you closer to your flat belly goal

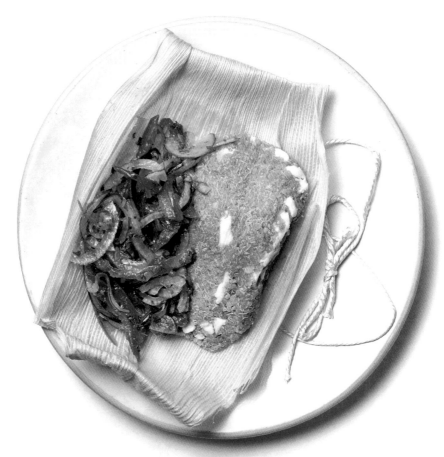

1: SUPER-CHARGING CORIANDER TAMALITO

SERVES 1 | CALS 614 | READY IN 45 MINS

*2 corn husks • 5ml olive oil
• 1 onion • 1 garlic clove
• 1 medium green chilli • 10
sprigs coriander, chopped
• Pinch cumin • 100g cooked
pearl quinoa • 30g feta • ½
red onion, chopped • ½ ripe
tomato • Juice of ½ lime*

Soak the corn husks in water
for 30 mins. Heat the oil in
a frying pan and sauté the
onion, garlic, chilli, most of
the coriander and the cumin
for 10 mins, then add the
quinoa. Season. Drain the corn
husks and place them on top
of each other. Position the

quinoa in the middle and add
the feta cheese to it. Wrap the
husks and mix into a parcel
using 40cm cotton string.
Cook the wrapped tamalito
in hot water for 5 mins. Serve
with salsa made with red
onion, tomato, the remainder
of the coriander and lime juice.

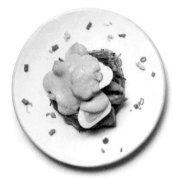

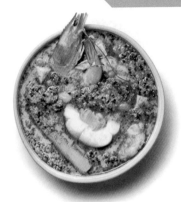

2: PROTEIN-PACK EGGS BENEDICTO
SERVES 1 | CALS 608 | READY IN 25 MINS

60g white and red quinoa • 20g flour • ½ egg, beaten • 250ml milk • 80g smoked trout • 2 asparagus spears • 40g spinach • 2 chillies, chopped • 1 egg

Boil the quinoa for 12 mins, drain, whisk in 10g flour, egg and 125ml milk. Shape into a muffin and fry until golden. Grill the trout; blanch the asparagus and spinach. Sauté the chillies, add remaining milk, 10g flour and whisk until thick. Place the greens and poached egg on the muffin.

3: FLAB-FIGHTING PRAWN CHOWDER
SERVES 1 | CALS 504 | READY IN 45 MINS

10 prawns (shells on) • 1 white onion, chopped • 1 garlic clove, crushed • 40g black quinoa • 1 potato, peeled • 10g broad beans • 10g peas • 1 egg • 2 tbsp double cream

Boil 8 prawns in 500ml water with onion, garlic, quinoa and potato for 30 mins. Add beans 10 mins before the end. Remove the prawns, peel and finely chop, then return to the liquid. Add the remaining prawns, peas and egg. Boil for 8 mins to poach the egg. Dress with cream.

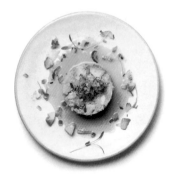

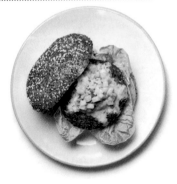

4: SLOW-BURN AVOCADO SALAD
SERVES 1 | CALS 428 | READY IN 15 MINS

75g quinoa • ¼ red chilli, chopped • 25g butter beans • Juice of ½ lime • 1 tsp olive oil • 3 coriander sprigs, chopped • ¼ avocado, chopped • ½ tsp honey • ⅛ red onion, diced • ¼ tomato, chopped

The fat in avocados doesn't head to your belly – it burns, slowly. Boil the quinoa for 12 mins, then drain and mix with the chilli, butter beans, lime juice, olive oil, coriander and avocado. Place the mixture in a bowl and pour in the honey, then mix in the onion and tomato.

5: CLEANSING QUINOA BURGER
SERVES 1 | CALS 721 | READY IN 1 HR

80g mixed quinoa • 1 onion, diced • ¼ green chilli, chopped • ¼ garlic clove, crushed • 1 egg, beaten • 20g plain flour • 2 tbsp breadcrumbs • 1 spelt roll • Lettuce • 2 tbsp yoghurt • 20g papaya, chopped • ¼ kiwi fruit, chopped

Boil the quinoa for 20 mins. Drain. Sauté onion, chilli and garlic in oil, then mix in egg and flour. Add the quinoa, shape into a patty, coat in breadcrumbs, chill for 30 mins and fry until golden. Put in the roll with lettuce, mix the remaining ingredients and place on top.

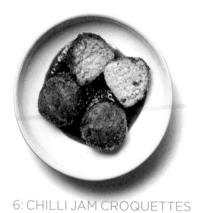

6: CHILLI JAM CROQUETTES
SERVES 1 | CALS 619 | READY IN 40 MINS

40g white quinoa · 1 onion, chopped · ¼ beaten egg · 2 tbsp Cheddar cheese · 2 sprigs coriander, chopped · 2 tbsp grated Parmesan · 2 tbsp breadcrumbs · 1 red chilli, chopped · 3 tbsp water · 3 tbsp sugar · 5 strawberries

Boil quinoa for 20 mins and fry onion in oil. Mix with egg, cheese, coriander and Parmesan. Form into 4 balls, coat in breadcrumbs and chill. Place the chilli, water, sugar and strawberries in a pan and reduce for 10 mins. Fry the balls in rapeseed oil until golden. Serve with the jam.

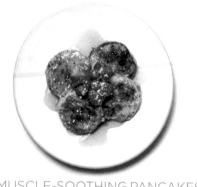

7: MUSCLE-SOOTHING PANCAKES
SERVES 1 | CALS 686 | READY IN 20 MINS

100g white quinoa · 20g plain flour · 2 tbsp milk · ½ egg, beaten · Pinch sugar · Pinch salt · 2 tbsp orange blossom honey · Pinch ground cinnamon · 40g berries

Perfect eats for post-gym recovery. Boil quinoa for 12 mins. Cool, then whisk in a bowl with the plain flour, milk, egg, 2 tbsp water, salt and sugar. Fry in a drop of olive oil until the pancake is golden on each side. Serve with the honey, sprinkled with cinnamon and berries.

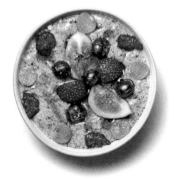

8: PERUVIAN POWER PORRIDGE
SERVES 1 | CALS 532 | READY IN 15 MINS

70g cooked quinoa · 40g cooked amaranth · 125ml quinoa milk · 4 tbsp honey · 10 blueberries · 4 strawberries · 5 goldenberries · 1 fig

Mix quinoa and amaranth together with quinoa milk and half the honey, bring to the boil and gently simmer for 10 mins. Once the mixture becomes creamy, serve in a bowl with the fig, strawberries, goldenberries, blueberries, and the remaining honey. Let your day begin.

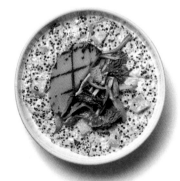

9: CREAMY SQUASH QUINOTTO
SERVES 1 | CALS 425 | READY IN 25 MINS

40g mixed quinoa · 60g squash, diced · ½ onion, chopped · ¼ garlic clove, crushed · 100g wild mushrooms · 125ml crème fraîche · 2 tbsp grated Parmesan

This is guilt-free comfort food. Boil squash and quinoa for 15 mins. Drain. Sauté onion and garlic for 5 mins. Add the mushrooms for 1 min, then the quinoa and squash mixture. Season and stir in the crème fraîche. Top with Parmesan, cooked wild mushrooms and a slice of roasted squash.

10: BELLY-SLIMMING LUCUMA MOUSSE
SERVES 1 | CALS 376 | READY IN 1 HR 40 MINS

10g flour • 10g cooked quinoa • 10g butter • 2 egg whites • 2 tbsp honey • Juice of 1 lemon • 2 tbsp xylitol • 4 tbsp lucuma powder • Kiwi fruit slices

If you have a sweet tooth, you'll love this low-carb Peruvian superfruit. Preheat the oven to 170°C. Mix the flour, quinoa, butter, 1 whisked egg white and honey. Put in the freezer for 20 mins, remove, then roll thinly. Bake for 5 mins, then let it cool over the end of a glass to make a basket shape. Whisk 1 egg white until stiff and add one half to the lemon juice and xylitol. Mix the lucuma powder with the other half. Fold the lemon mix into this and put in the fridge for 1 hour. Serve in the biscuit basket with the kiwi.

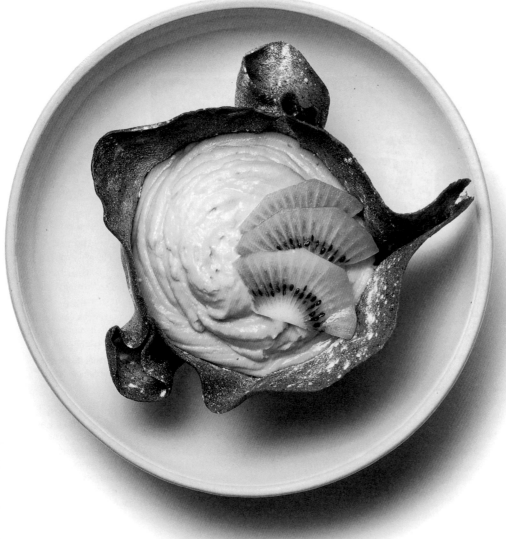

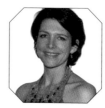

MY FLAT BELLY DIARY:

Thomasina Miers

As the founder of Wahaca Mexican restaurants, Thomasina Miers is constantly thinking about food. How does she manage to keep temptation at bay?

MONDAY

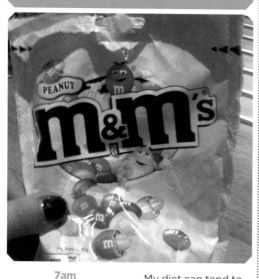

7am
Earl Grey tea

8am
Home-made muesli with nuts, oats and bran

1:30pm
Toast with taramasalata

3pm
Kale sautéed with chilli and a fried egg

8:30pm
M&Ms and a herbal tea

My diet can tend to be quite erratic. I take an iron supplement every day because I became anaemic after having my second child, but I've been quite bad at adjusting my diet since then. I try to smuggle in leafy green vegetables and fresh fruit wherever I can.

TUESDAY

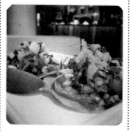

8am
Toast with peanut butter, yoghurt with baked rhubarb

11am-3pm
Recipe-testing ceviche with corn and beans

4pm
Tomato salad with mint tea

8:30pm
Asparagus salad with leftover ceviche

I eat lots of vegetables on weekdays. It's not a conscious thing to just eat meat at the weekend, but I only visit the butcher on Saturdays and I never buy meat from the supermarket.

WEDNESDAY

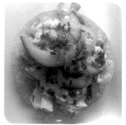

8am
A pear

11am
Flat white coffee

2pm
Smoked herring tostada

3-6pm
Tasting ceviche, Caesar salad, crab and chorizo empanadas

9:30pm
Lemongrass, mint and camomile tea

I find tea is a real cure-all. I have Earl Grey to wake me up and give me energy in the morning and drink this lemon grass, mint and camomile mix before bed because it's so calming.

AS TOLD TO: AMELIA JEAN JONES. PHOTOGRAPHY: GETTY IMAGES. CHILLI NOTES RECIPES TO WARM THE HEART (NOT BURN THE TONGUE)

THURSDAY	FRIDAY	SATURDAY	SUNDAY

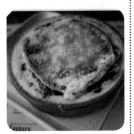 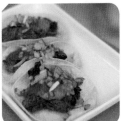 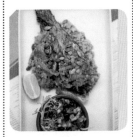 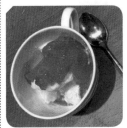

THURSDAY

7am
Earl Grey tea

8am
Rhubarb and yoghurt

1:30pm
Tasting fish tacos and corn lasagne with two glasses of mescal liquor

9pm
Prawn and tomato curry, rice and peas

11pm
Camomile tea

I'm a professional eater, but feeling guilty about what you eat is so counter-productive. It's why people have unhealthy attitudes to food. Variation and moderation are key.

FRIDAY

8am
Tea and toast with Marmite

11am
Chorizo quesadilla

1pm
Chicken tacos with beans, rice and vegetables

8:30pm
Beetroot soup

9pm
Apple purée and ice cream

Sometimes I'm too tired to cook a full meal. We grow vegetables in our back garden so I take fresh produce and make something wholesome like beetroot soup.

SATURDAY

8am
Earl Grey tea

9am
Toast and yoghurt with cereal

1pm
Grilled fish with guacamole, refried beans, tacos and a quesadilla

8pm
Chocolate ice-cream and peanut M&Ms

Since my second child was born a year ago, I haven't done any exercise except cycling 12 miles to work each day. My new goal is to play tennis; I need that competitive element.

SUNDAY

8:30am
An apple

9:30am
Coffee with cream

1pm
Fish pie, mashed potatoes and broccoli

1:30pm
Yoghurt and baked rhubarb

8:30pm
Chilli kale with a fried egg

My grandmother was a model and very slim, but she always ate butter on toast. I never believed that low-fat food was good for you and now scientists agree.

THE EXPERT VERDICT

Our nutritionist Dr Christy Fergusson gives her feedback: "You can tell that Thomasina takes a keen interest in nutrition. Her herbal tea habit keeps her hydrated, while anything with chilli in it boosts metabolism. Studies also show capsaicin – the stuff that makes chillis hot – helps to protect your body from cancer.

"She eats her biggest meals at lunch, which is great, but her diet lacks routine later because she's so busy. Obviously, a lot depends on how healthy the foods are that she's tasting at work.

"The variety of fish she eats provides protein and healthy fats to fuel her busy days, while green vegetables are packed with immunity-boosting antioxidants. However, Thomasina often only has a cup of tea, yoghurt or fruit in the morning.

"A larger, more balanced breakfast of low-GI carbs, protein and essential fats – such as chia seeds with coconut yoghurt and raspberries, for example – would get her off to a better start."

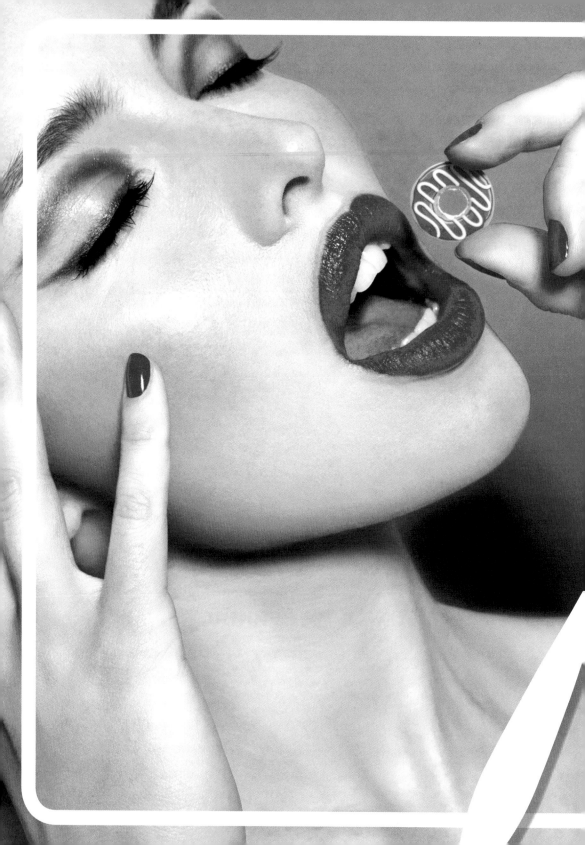

SNACKS AND TREATS

Food is supposed to be joyful: no day should be without a treat. Smart snacking curbs cravings and gives your body and mind the nourishment they need. That's why we've come up with a collection of the best (and most delicious) treats for you to indulge in. And if that isn't enough to make you turn the page, many of these little gems have less than 100 calories. Yum!

Tuna Indulgence Canapés

This recipe is as simple as it is delicious. Serve up these tiny treats to impress your guests

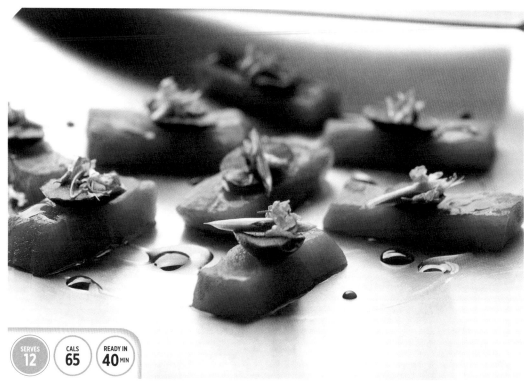

SERVES 12 **CALS 65** **READY IN 40 MIN**

Tuna is a 'meaty' protein-rich fish, so it's great for filling you up without being too calorific. 'Cooking' the meat with lime juice and salt will help it retain more of its protein value than conventional, heat-based methods. Researchers at the Virginia Polytechnic Institute recently showed that the flavanols in dark chocolate may prevent weight gain and help lower blood sugar levels. Not too shabby!

INGREDIENTS

- *300g/11oz fresh tuna, skin removed and cut into 12 pieces*
- *2 tbsp balsamic vinegar*
- *Juice of half a lime*
- *3 tbsp extra virgin olive oil*
- *30g/1oz plain (dark) chocolate, 85-90% cocoa solids, cut into small pieces*
- *Rosemary flowers*

METHOD

1 First, put the tuna pieces in a large bowl. Now toss with the vinegar, lime juice, oil and a pinch of salt; keep it nice and gentle. Transfer to the fridge to chill for 30 mins (you too, preferably with a nice big glass of something).

2 Back with us? OK, now season the tuna with salt and pepper and arrange just so on a serving dish.

3 For your final flourish, arrange the chocolate and rosemary flowers artfully on top of each piece and place on your finest bit of china.

Mini Pear Tarts

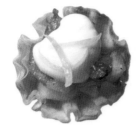

SERVES 18

CALS 43

READY IN 110 MIN

4 tsp unsalted butter • 2 pears, peeled, cored and diced into ½-inch cubes • 1 tbsp fresh lemon juice • 2½ tsp brown sugar • Pinch salt • 4 tsp plain low-fat Greek yoghurt • 18 mini Filo pastry tarts

1 The yoghurt and fruit in these tiny treats really do make small into beautiful. Melt butter in a large pan over a low heat. Add pears, 2 tbsp of the brown sugar, lemon juice and the salt. Stir gently until the pears are tender but not falling apart. Mix the yoghurt with the remaining sugar.

2 Spoon the pear mixture into the tart cases – about 1 tbsp for each one. Top each tart case with ½ tsp of the yoghurt mixture.

Chocolate Surprise

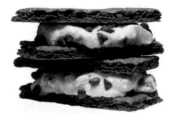

SERVES 8

CALS 120

READY IN 63 MIN

65g low-fat ricotta • 1½ tbsp orange marmalade • 1 tbsp sugar • 1 tbsp mini plain chocolate chips • 16 chocolate wafers (or you could also use ginger thins)

1 Tangy flavour and low-fat ricotta make little servings go a long way. Stir the ricotta, sugar, marmalade and chocolate chips in a small bowl until combined.

2 Place 8 of the wafers on a baking sheet, and top them with a generous tablespoon of the ricotta mixture.

3 Top with the remaining wafers and freeze for about an hour until set. Serve frozen.

Mini Red Cupcakes

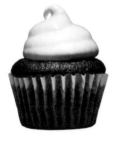

SERVES 48

CALS 34

READY IN 110 MIN

Half a box red velvet cake mix • 120ml water • 3 tbsp Bramley apple sauce (unsweetened) • 1 large egg, plus 1 egg white • 100g Marshmallow Fluff (find it in some supermarkets like Asda)

1 A tiny treat with an apple twist. Preheat oven to 170°C. Combine the cake mix, water, apple sauce, egg and egg white in a large bowl, and beat until smooth. Spoon the mix into mini cupcake cases in a tin and bake for 15 to 17 mins.

2 Let cool for 1 min in the pan, then on a wire rack. Use a plastic bag with a corner snipped off to pipe a blob of Marshmallow Fluff on top.

Spiced Pudding

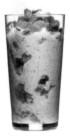

SERVES 8

CALS 80

READY IN 4 MIN

1 can Ambrosia Low Fat Rice Pudding • ¼ tsp ground cardamom • ¼ tsp ground cinnamon • 40g dried apricots, chopped • 40g pistachios, chopped

1 A comfortingly warm, slow-burn pudding with appetite-squishing cinnamon. Get spicy. Decant the rice pudding into a non-stick pan and heat it on the hob. After a minute or two, stir in the spices and half the apricots and nuts.

2 When heated through, divide the mixture between eight tall shot glasses and sprinkle with the remaining apricots and pistachios.

Chocolate & Rosemary Biscuits

It might sound like a strange combo, but trust us, these two ingredients get along perfectly

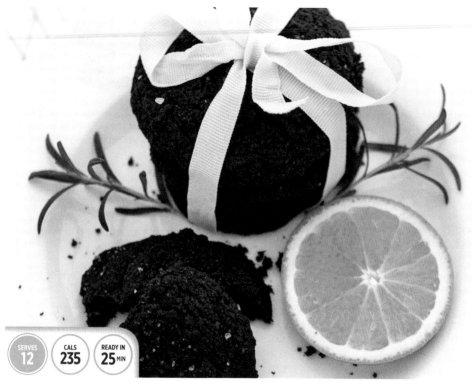

SERVES 12   **CALS** 235   **READY IN** 25 MIN

Spelt flour has 5 per cent more vitamin B3 than normal white flour, which boosts energy and is easier to digest. Plus, it's low-GI, so will leave you feeling satisfied after just one biscuit (handy as they have a relatively high saturated fat content). Add the rosemary – a proven indigestion cure – and these might just be the best way to soothe a bloated stomach.

INGREDIENTS
- 150g spelt flour
- 250g unsalted butter
- 2 sprigs rosemary, finely chopped
- Zest of 1 orange
- 100g 70% dark chocolate
- 1 tsp baking powder
- 1 tsp bicarb of soda
- ½ tsp salt
- 175g raw sugar
- 3 free-range eggs
- 3 tbsp maple syrup
- ½ tbsp vanilla extract
- Coarse sea salt

METHOD

1 Preheat the oven to 200°C, then line a baking sheet with parchment paper. Sift the flour into a bowl with the baking powder, bicarb and salt.

2 Whack the butter and sugar in a separate bowl and beat until pale and light. Add the eggs one at a time then whisk in the vanilla and maple syrup. Add the dry ingredients in three batches, stirring well after each addition. Add the rosemary, orange zest and chocolate, then give it one last stir – use those biceps!

3 Drop 2 tbsp of biscuit dough on to the prepared tray, leaving 2in between each biscuit. Sprinkle each one with a little salt.

4 Place the tray on the middle shelf and bake for 10 mins. Remove from the oven. Best eaten when slightly warm and chewy. Heaven.

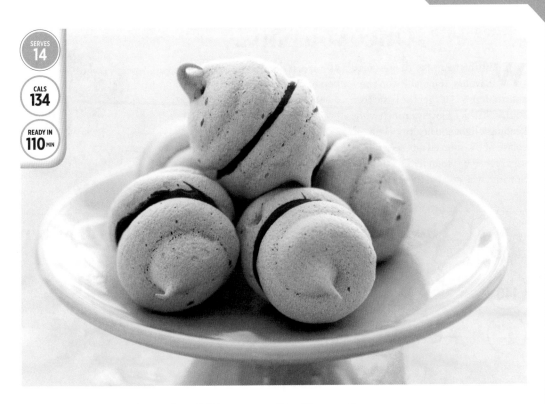

SERVES
14

CALS
134

READY IN
110 MIN

Mini Choc Meringues

These treats are small but perfectly formed. Don't worry, we won't judge you for scoffing

Augustus Gloop and women across the land have at least one thing in common (that we know of) – we all love a good bit of chocolate. If you're getting that nagging impulse to pop to the newsagent, try the flat belly option – a hazelnut chocolate spread contains appetite-regulating protein and will put the brakes on that post-binge blood sugar spike. Sinful? Fat chance.

INGREDIENTS
- 2 egg whites
- 110g caster sugar
- 3-4 tbsp low fat, sugar-free chocolate hazelnut spread (£3.85, mydukandietshop.co.uk)

METHOD

1 Heat the oven to its lowest setting. Line a large baking tray with non-stick paper.

2 Whisk the egg whites until soft peaks form. Gradually whisk in the sugar until stiff and glossy. When baking meringues or cakes, don't use eggs straight from the fridge. The coiled proteins in egg whites are more relaxed at room temperature, so they can be beaten to a foam more easily.

3 Spoon 28 small portions on to a baking tray. Cook for 1-2 hours, until the meringues feel crisp and lift off the paper easily. Switch off the oven and leave them inside to cool, ideally overnight, for a crunchy shell and gooey centre.

4 Spread the meringues with generous helpings of chocolate spread, then sandwich them together.

Once you pop...

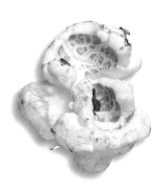

With this many 150-calories-max flavours, you really won't be able to stop. So let's get the basic corn started. "To get a lovely crunch while keeping it light and healthy, use a splash of UK-sourced rapeseed oil," says Propercorn founder Cassandra Stavrou, who created these recipes.

1 Pour just enough oil into a large pan to cover the base. Place on a high heat, add 100g of popcorn kernels and mix with a wooden spoon to coat evenly with oil.

2 Put on the lid and leave it until you hear a pop. Shake every 20 seconds till the pops slow to every 3 seconds. Remove from the heat.

The Dark Side

SERVES **4**

CALS **140**

READY IN **2** MIN

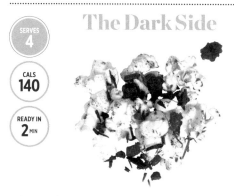

1 tbsp unsalted butter, melted · 25g dark chocolate, grated · 35g freeze-dried raspberries

Pour the butter over the popcorn, then mix in the chocolate and chopped raspberries.

Some Like It Hotter

SERVES **4**

CALS **121**

READY IN **3** MIN

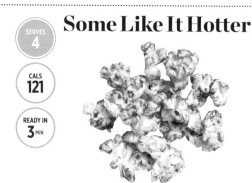

1 tbsp coconut oil · 1 tsp ground cumin seeds · Pinch each of curry powder, turmeric and garlic powder

Melt coconut oil in a small pan, pour it on the popcorn and stir in the seeds and spices.

Nut Enough

SERVES **4**

CALS **149**

READY IN **2** MIN

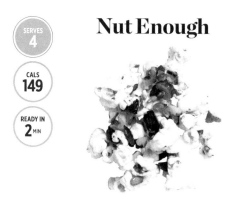

2 tbsp agave nectar ·20g pumpkin and sunflower seeds · Handful of dried cranberries · 20g mixed nuts

Drizzle the popcorn with the agave nectar, then mix in seeds, berries and chopped nuts.

The Big Chilli

SERVES **4**

CALS **105**

READY IN **2** MIN

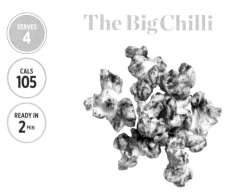

1 tbsp olive oil · 1tsp cumin · 1 tsp chilli powder (or to taste) · Dried zest from 2 limes · Pinch of salt

Splash the oil over the popcorn, then mix in all the other ingredients and give it a shake.

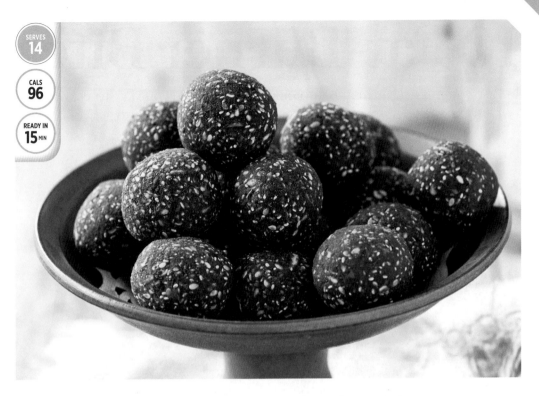

SERVES 14

CALS 96

READY IN 15 MIN

Rejuvenating Petits Fours

Easy to make and even easier to eat, get to work on these guilt-free chocolate truffles

This recipe's not just a fat-burner; it's a beauty booster too. The raw cacao revs up your metabolism to attack fatty deposits in your body, plus it boosts circulation to help zap dark eye circles. Oh, and the whizzing up of the chia seeds that this recipe calls for makes them more easily absorbed by your body – so you'll reap even more benefits from their skin-plumping omega-3. Looking good.

INGREDIENTS
- 50ml coconut milk
- 125g nut butter (any)
- 30g ground cacao
- 60g chia seeds
- 75g sesame seeds
- 75g pumpkin seeds
- 75g sunflower seeds
- 75g coconut flour
- 2 tbsp rice malt syrup

METHOD

1 You won't believe how easy this one is. Simply place all the ingredients in a blender and pulse until smooth.

2 Remove 1 tbsp of the mix and roll it to form a small ball. Repeat until you've used up all the mix.

3 Store the truffles in an airtight container; they'll keep in the fridge for two weeks, or for three months in the freezer. Assuming they haven't all been devoured within seconds, that is.

10 Fat-Burner Bites

In case you missed the memo, protein is kryptonite to your fat stores, which is why we've whipped up some new portable, snackable ways to get your fill…

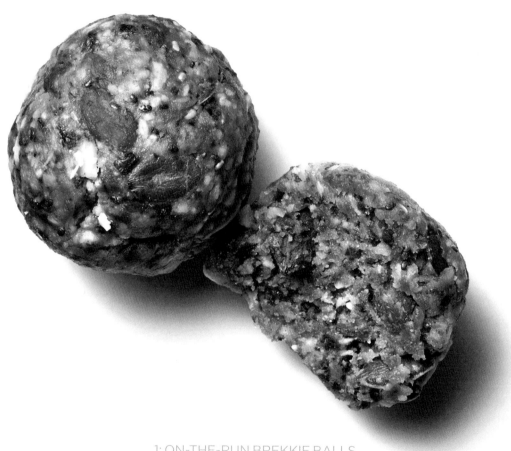

1: ON-THE-RUN BREKKIE BALLS
MAKES 7 | 217 CALS | 8.2G PROTEIN | READY IN 30 MINS

50g almonds · 25g hazelnuts · 40g brown rice protein · 40g cranberries · 10g each goji berries and chia, hemp, sunflower and pumpkin seeds · 35g coconut oil · 30g maple syrup · 1 tsp vanilla extract

Ready? Get your food processor out and start by blitzing together the almonds, roasted hazelnuts and rice protein. Set aside. Next, whizz the cranberries. Combine with the nuts, goji berries and seeds. Melt the coconut oil, add the syrup and vanilla and stir into the fruit and nuts. Pop in the fridge for 20 mins, then roll into balls. Boom. Chia seeds expand in your stomach, while pumpkin seeds are packed with fibre, so they'll keep you full till lunch. Just don't eat the lot.

THE GOOD LIFE EATERY, 59 SLOANE AVENUE, LONDON SW3 3DH; GOODLIFEEATERY.COM. NUTRITIONAL ANALYSIS: RUTH REYNOLDS.

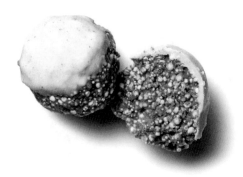

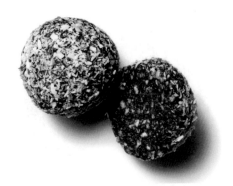

2: ANY TIME PEANUT BUTTER BALLS
MAKES 7 | 175 CALS | 7.5G PROTEIN
READY IN 30 MINS

75g peanut butter • 20g coconut oil • 10g agave nectar • 5g Madagascar vanilla • 30g brown rice protein • 35g puffed quinoa • 30g amaranth, toasted • 50g organic vegan white chocolate

Combine the peanut butter, coconut oil, agave and vanilla. Melt the mixture gently over a bowl of hot water. Add the rice protein, quinoa and amaranth. Mix well, then pop in the fridge for 15 mins and roll into balls. Melt the chocolate and dip the tops in, allow to harden then serve.

3: MORNING GLORY ENERGY BALLS
MAKES 10 | 150 CALS | 4G PROTEIN
READY IN 10 MINS

70g Brazil nuts • 30g sunflower seeds • 120g dried apple • 10g ashwagandha • 1 tsp spirulina • 40g hemp protein • 2 tsp acai powder • ½ banana • 30g honey • 20g coconut oil • Desiccated coconut

In a blender, blitz the Brazil nuts and sunflower seeds and set aside. Then whizz up the apple, ashwagandha (a powdered herb), spirulina, hemp, acai, banana and honey then mix in the nuts and melted coconut oil. Roll into balls and cover in the coconut.

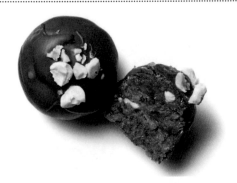

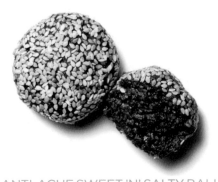

4: PRE-GYM 'FAUX-RERO ROCHERS'
MAKES 11 | 423 CALS | 7.3G PROTEIN
READY IN 20 MINS

225g dates • 50g hazelnut butter • 30g brown rice protein • 10g raw maca powder • 20g maple syrup • 30g coconut oil • 50g hazelnuts • 500g vegan dark chocolate

Whizz up the dates, add the butter, rice protein, maca and syrup and blitz. Stir in the coconut oil and refrigerate until hard. Roll into balls. Roast 11 hazelnuts and push one into the centre. Coat in melted chocolate twice, allowing each layer to cool. Top with crushed hazelnuts.

5: ANTI-ACHE SWEET 'N' SALTY BALLS
MAKES 8 | 134 CALS | 8.1G PROTEIN
READY IN 20 MINS

30g pecans • 20g dates, chopped • 70g hazelnut butter • 40g tahini • 30g brown rice protein • 7g raw cacao powder • 25g raw honey • 1 tsp cinnamon • 20g coconut oil • 30g sesame seeds

The gym-goer's friend. Whizz up the pecans and dates. Add the hazelnut butter, tahini, rice protein, cacao, honey and cinnamon. Blitz the lot until smooth then pour in the melted coconut oil and whizz again quickly. Roll into balls and coat with sesame.

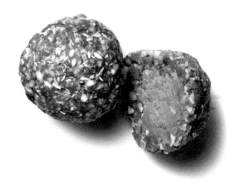

6: POST-WORKOUT VITAMIN C BALLS
**MAKES 8 | 185 CALS | 6.9G PROTEIN
READY IN 10 MINS†**

150g dried apricot • Zest of 1 lemon • Juice of ½ lemon • 10g baobab powder • 100g almonds • 30g organic brown rice protein • 30g maple syrup • 15g coconut oil, melted • 30g coconut flakes

Baobab is your high-fibre, low calorie hero. Blitz 100g apricots with lemon zest, juice and baobab. Roll into balls and refrigerate. Whizz up the rice protein, almonds, rest of the apricots and syrup, then mix in the coconut oil and flakes. Roll each ball in the crust and refrigerate for an hour.

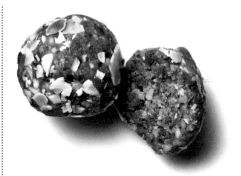

7: METABOLISM-REVVING FIREBALLS
**MAKES 9 | 191 CALS | 8.6G PROTEIN
READY IN 10 MINS**

100g almonds • 50g cranberries • Zest of 1 orange and 1 lemon • 40g brown rice protein powder • 5g acai powder • 3g cayenne pepper • 25g coconut oil • 50g goji berries (pre-soaked in water) • 50g roasted flaked almonds

Cayenne, acai and goji join forces to stoke your body's furnace. Blitz the almonds, add cranberries, orange and lemon zest, rice protein, acai and cayenne until evenly blitzed. Add the melted coconut oil and fold in the goji berries. Roll into balls and press them in the flaked almonds.

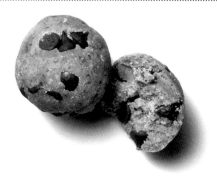

8: AFTER-DINNER COOKIE BALLS
**MAKES 8 | 80 CALS | 4G PROTEIN
READY IN 15 MINS**

25g brown rice protein • 15g coconut sugar • 25g coconut flour • 15g coconut oil • 30g almond butter • 50ml almond milk • 5g vanilla extract • 30g raw cacao nibs

Hidden protein defeats the sugar spike. Whizz up the rice protein, coconut sugar and coconut flour. Add the melted coconut oil, almond butter, almond milk, vanilla and a pinch of salt and blitz. Fold in the cacao nibs. Roll into balls with damp hands to keep them from falling apart.

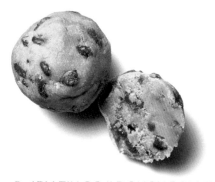

9: 4PM FIX GOJI DOUGH BALLS
**MAKES 7 | 157 CALS | 6.6G PROTEIN
READY IN 15 MINS**

30g xylitol • 90g sunflower spread, softened • 80g gluten-free flour • 40g brown rice protein • 10g vanilla extract • 50g goji berries

Put down the cookie jar! Blitz the xylitol until it's powdery like icing sugar. In a separate bowl, whisk the sunflower spread until light and fluffy. Slowly whisk in the flour, rice protein, vanilla extract and a pinch of salt. Gently fold in the goji berries. Roll into balls to avoid them breaking.

10: GYM-FUELLING AVO-COCO BON BONS
MAKES 20 | 142 CALS | 3.5G PROTEIN | READY IN 20 MINS

1 medium avocado · 2 bananas · 300g coconut cream · 40g raw honey · 50g brown rice protein · 45g cacao nibs · 200g vegan dark chocolate, melted

Mash the avocado, banana, coconut cream, honey and rice protein until smooth. Stir in 45g of the cacao nibs, keeping 5g for the topping. Freeze this mixture, then use an ice cream scoop to shape it into balls. Melt the chocolate, then roll the balls in it. Finally, top them with crushed cacao nibs. Get them while they're, er, cold. Avocado and bananas are packed with potassium – vital for healthy muscles. Chow down before a cardio session and give 'em hell.

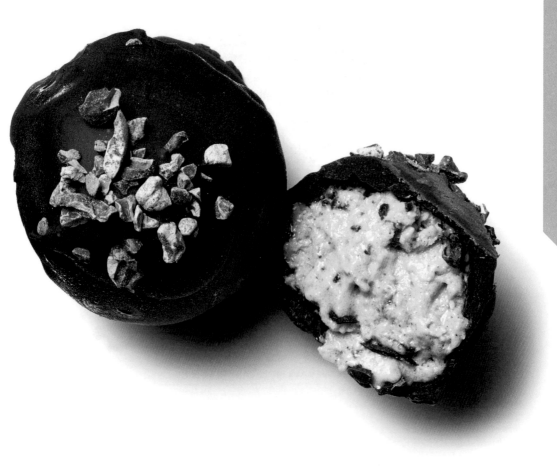

10 Slimful Bakes

How can you have a sweet treat without damaging your diet? Get clever with ingredients. Skinny Bakery founder Mariella Crosthwait shows us how

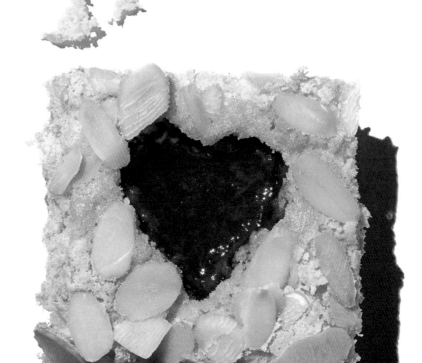

1: LOW-SUGAR CHERRY BAKEWELL

SERVES 9 | CALS 148 | READY IN 50 MINS

3 large eggs • 75g fructose • 75g xylitol • 150g plain flour, sifted • 1 tsp vanilla essence • 15g flaked almonds • 150g low-sugar cherry jam

Prepped for some serious baking? Start by preheating the oven to 180°C. Whisk the eggs with the fructose and xylitol for 10 mins. Fold in the flour, then the vanilla and 1 tbsp water. Divide into two greased and lined 9in x 9in tins. Sprinkle one with flaked almonds. Bake both for 20 mins. Cut nine hearts out of the almond layer. Mix the jam with 50ml warm water, then spread over the plain layer. Place the almond layer on top, then slice into 3in x 3in squares and serve. Cherry, cherry good.

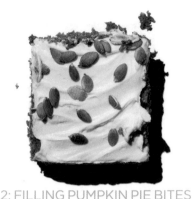

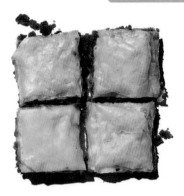

2: FILLING PUMPKIN PIE BITES
SERVES 9 | CALS 151 | READY IN 50 MINS

3 eggs • 80g fructose • Almond essence • Zest 1 orange • 130g grated pumpkin • 1 tsp corn oil • 2 tbsp stevia • 2 tbsp fructose • 100g flour • 1 tsp each bicarb soda & baking powder • 1½ tsp cinnamon • ½ tsp cream of tartar • 175g cream cheese

Preheat oven to 170°C. Mix yolks, fructose, stevia, zest, pumpkin, oil, almond and 2 tbsp water. Separately, mix flour, bicarb, baking powder and cinnamon. Whisk egg whites with tartar until stiff. Combine mixes, then fold in whites. Bake for 30 mins. Cool. Top with cream cheese and seeds.

3: SUGAR-FREE BAKLAVA
SERVES 9 | CALS 145 | READY IN 1 HR

18 sheets filo pastry • Light oil spray • 225g chestnuts, chopped • 25g xylitol • 1 tsp cinnamon • 90g xylitol • 40g honey • 2 tbsp orange blossom water • 100ml water

Preheat oven to 170°C. Fill a baking tray with half the filo pastry sprayed with oil. Mix chestnuts, xylitol and cinnamon and spread over. Top with the rest of the filo and prick with a knife. Bake for 40 mins, then heat rest of ingredients and water for 10-15 mins and drizzle over. Slice.

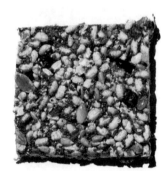

4: FULL TUMMY CHIA SEED BARS
SERVES 9 | CALS 139 | READY IN 10 MINS†

44g wholegrain puffed rice • ½ tsp dried ginger • ½ tsp cardamom • 60g chia seeds • 60g pumpkin seeds, sunflower seeds, linseeds, dried apricots, dried cranberries and blueberries • 40g almond butter • 50g honey • 60g xylitol

Chia seed is the enemy of hunger and loaded with antioxidants. Start by mixing the dry ingredients, then heat the almond butter, honey and xylitol until well dissolved, then stir in. Mix and press into a non-stick 9in x 9in tin, refrigerate overnight then cut into 9 squares.

5: LOW-GUILT CHOCOLATE BROWNIE
SERVES 9 | CALS 191 | READY IN 35 MINS

85g gluten-free flour • Pinch xanthan gum • 25g cocoa powder • ¼ tsp bicarb soda • 150g fructose • 25g seed mix • 1 egg • 80g light mayo • ½ tsp vanilla extract • 50g low-fat yoghurt • 50g dark chocolate, melted

Preheat the oven to 180°C. Mix the dry ingredients, then the wet ones, with 2 tbsp water. Bake for 25 mins in a non-stick 9in x 9in tray. It's cooked when it pulls away from the edges (i.e. you don't get a gooey fork when testing). Cut into 9 squares when cool. Choc around the clock.

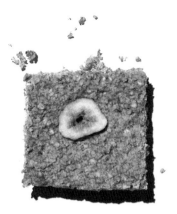

6: GLUTEN-FREE BANANA FLAPJACK

SERVES 9 | CALS 164 | READY IN 35 MINS

50g fructose · 25g unsalted butter · 25g agave syrup · 50g gluten-free flour · ½ tsp bicarb soda · ½ tsp baking powder · 200g porridge oats · Pinch xanthan gum · 140g ripe banana, puréed

The slow-burn snack. Preheat oven to 170°C. Melt fructose, butter and agave syrup in a pan. Mix flour, bicarb, baking powder, oats and xanthan gum and add in. Stir in puréed banana with 2 tbsp cold water. Bake in a non-stick 9in x 9in tray for 20 mins. Cut when cooled.

7: TAKE-ANYWHERE TIRAMISU

SERVES 9 | CALS 114 | READY IN 20 MINS†

50g egg whites · 10g fructose · 250g light cream cheese · 20ml marsala wine · 3 tsp stevia · 150g sponge fingers · 100ml strong coffee · 2 tsp cocoa powder · 10g dark chocolate, grated

Whisk whites to stiff peaks, add fructose until it's glossy. Separately, blend the cream cheese with the marsala and stevia. Dip sponge fingers in coffee and layer in a tray. Spread cream over the fingers, dust with cocoa and chocolate. Refrigerate overnight, cut into squares and enjoy.

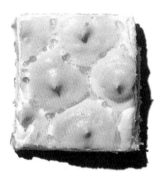

8: LOW-CALORIE LEMON MERINGUE

SERVES 9 | CALS 117 | READY IN 1 HR†

15g xylitol · Juice and zest of 2 lemons · 2 eggs, beaten · 100g trifle sponges, halved · 6 egg whites · ¼ tsp cream of tartar · 100g sugar

Dissolve xylitol in juice over a low heat. Remove, whisk in eggs, add zest then heat to thicken. Put half the curd in a tin, then sponge, then rest of curd. Refrigerate overnight. Set oven to 160°C. Whisk whites with cream of tartar until stiff. Fold in sugar, pipe onto base and bake for 35 mins.

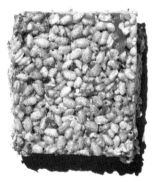

9: LOW-FAT PEANUT BUTTER BAR

SERVES 9 | CALS 175 | READY IN 20 MINS†

100g caster sugar · 85g honey · 95g reduced-fat peanut butter · 95g puffed wholegrain rice

Melt caster sugar, honey and peanut butter in a pan. Stir the puffed rice into the mixture, then press into a 9in x 9in non-stick baking tray. We hope you're not hungry... this one needs to go in the fridge overnight. The next morning, cut into squares. Perfect for the gym bag.

10: FLAT BELLY FESTIVE TREAT
SERVES 9 | CALS 127 | READY IN 45 MINS†

80g mixed fruit and peel
• 2 tbsp rum • 3 eggs • 25g
honey • 25g fructose • 1 tsp oil
• 100g flour • 1 tsp bicarb soda
• 1 tsp baking powder • 1½ tsp
mixed spice • ¼ tsp cream of
tartar • 1 tbsp reduced-sugar
marmalade • Royal icing

Preheat oven to 170°C. Soak the fruit in rum and 3 tbsp water for a few hours to soften. Separate eggs and whisk the yolks, honey, fructose, fruits and oil. Separately, mix the flour, bicarb, baking powder and spice. Whisk whites with cream of tartar until stiff. Stir the flour into yolks, then fold in egg whites. Bake in a tray for 25 mins. Microwave the marmalade with 1 tbsp boiling water for 30 seconds and spread over the hot bake. Cool, roll out the icing and cut out nine stars. Slice into squares and top with a star.

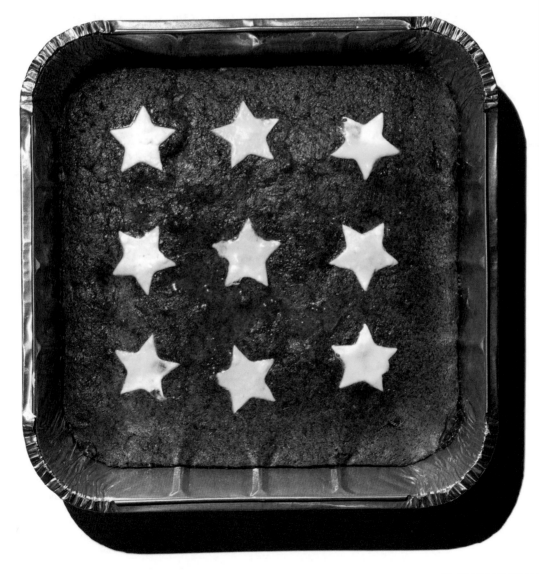

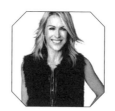

MY FLAT BELLY DIARY:

Lorna Jane Clarkson

Ms Clarkson is a living advert for Lorna Jane, Australia's biggest fitnesswear brand. Let's head Down Under to find out how she stays Lycra-ready

MONDAY

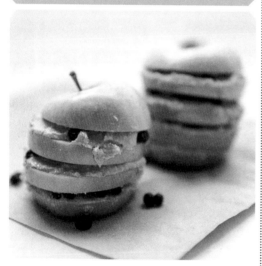

6am
Oats with banana and berries

10am
Apple with almond butter

1:30pm
Chicken and kale salad with carrot, radish and pepper

7pm
Lentil soup with broccoli, green beans, courgette and spinach

I tend to kick off most of my mornings with stretches on my yoga mat, then later on I meet with my trainer to go through an hour-long strength-building session. I love resistance training; it's perfect for raising my energy levels and helps to prevent injuries, too.

TUESDAY

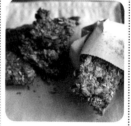

7:30am
Chocolate whey protein, berries, Greek yoghurt and spinach smoothie

1pm
Brussels sprout salad with lemon chicken

4pm
Home-made granola bar

7:30pm
Baked fish with olives and sweet potato and tomato salad

I like to exercise first thing to stay motivated for the rest of the day. Fitting in a daily workout is non-negotiable, as is eating well – making my own healthy snacks also helps.

WEDNESDAY

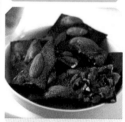

6am
Oats with cacao nibs and pumpkin seeds

11am
Green smoothie with ginger

1:30pm
Roast beetroot and lentil salad

6:30pm
Chicken, pear and goat's cheese salad

7:30pm
Home-made nut chocolate

Surrounding yourself with people who encourage you is the best way to boost willpower. Once a week, I take my home-made nut chocolate on a 5K walk with a friend.

AS TOLD TO: AMELIA JEAN JONES

THURSDAY

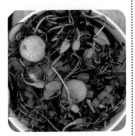

7:30am
Chocolate whey protein, banana and coconut water smoothie

10am
A shot of 2 tsp bee pollen mixed with 2 tsp coconut oil

1:30pm
Radish, sprout and red cabbage salad

7:30pm
Roast lamb with kale pesto and baby carrots

Every so often, I spend an hour dry body brushing before a yoga and meditation session. The vigorous motion eases muscle soreness. It's definitely worth the time.

FRIDAY

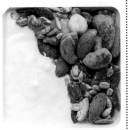

6am
Oats soaked in filtered water with cacao, coconut flakes and blueberries

10:30am
Greek yoghurt with home-made spiced nut mix

1:30pm
Scallop and asparagus salad

6:30pm
Moroccan chicken tagine with black rice

I switch my workouts to keep things exciting. My new favourite is Cardio Barre – a fun dance class I do three times a week that tones my bum, legs, core and arms.

SATURDAY

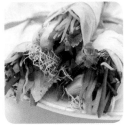

7am
Pepper, spinach, turmeric and tomato omelette

11am
Bee pollen & fresh fruit salad

2pm
Prawn rice paper rolls with raw vegetable crudités

7pm
Salmon with roast vegetables

7:30pm
Apple, berry and cacao crumble

I like to ease myself into the weekend with a good breakfast, a big cup of green tea and a good book to read. Then I'll grab my water bottle and hit the fitness trail for a hike.

SUNDAY

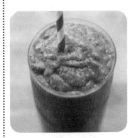

6:30am
Courgette, kale, banana, ginger and lemon smoothie

10am
Spinach and pepper frittata

1pm
Grilled chicken and broccoli salad

6:30pm
Omelette with chicken, pepper, kale, tomato, courgette and asparagus

When I go to my beach house at weekends, I always pack my running shoes. After a run on the sand, I'll swim in the Australian ocean – it sets me up for the week.

THE EXPERT VERDICT

Nutritionist Dr Christy Fergusson gives her feedback: "Lorna Jane's diet is great. It's packed with a wide variety of fresh, nutrient-dense foods. She eats every three to four hours – perfect for maintaining healthy blood-sugar levels, and she sticks with low-GI carbs such as sweet potato and oats.

"The bee pollen is a nutritious addition because it's packed with carbs, protein and B vitamins to keep her energy levels steady, while its enzymes aid digestion.

"Because some whey powders contain added sweeteners, the only suggestion I would make is to switch her chocolate whey protein powder to a more natural, plant-based protein powder such as hemp or brown rice powder, both of which have a full amino acid complex and are also gluten free.

"Her green smoothies are a smart addition because they're rich in nutrients but low in calories, so you get more bang for your meal-time buck."

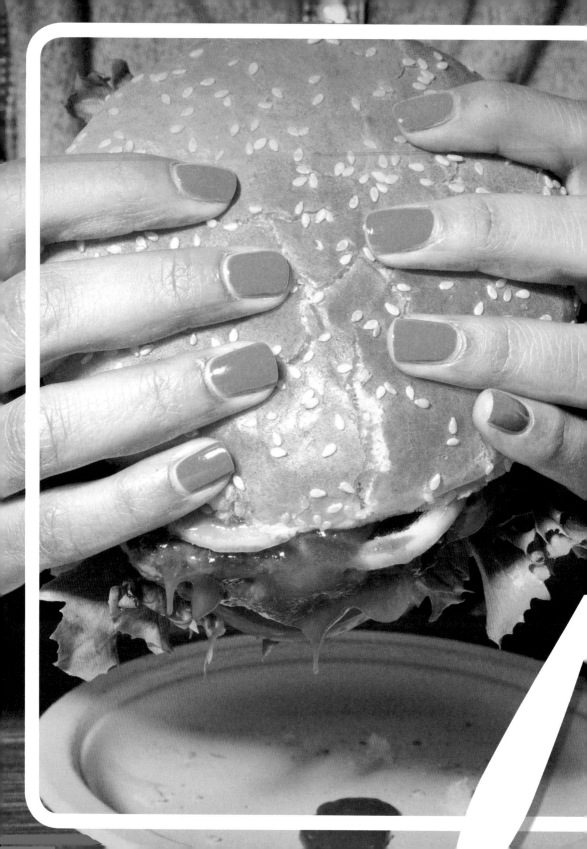

WINNING DINNERS

Tired? You're about to hit the flat belly danger zone. It's easy to give in and reach for the takeaway menu, but you're likely to end up plumping for a carb-heavy comforter that'll turn to fat while you sleep. We've put these tempting, easy-prep dishes together to help keep you fuller for longer and supercharge your metabolism as you slumber. No more night terrors, then.

Chilli Chicken & Mushroom Burger

No need to ban the barbecue! Choose the flat belly option and keep your licence to grill

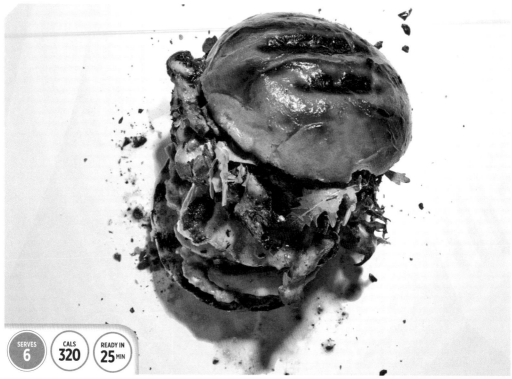

SERVES **6** CALS **320** READY IN **25** MIN

Chillies are rich in capsaicin, which can increase your metabolism by 23 per cent for up to three hours after eating. Chicken burgers have around 70 per cent less fat than beef burgers and thighs are higher in protein than mince, so are a better option. With a combination of protein and chillies, this burger is sure to keep you feeling fuller for longer.

INGREDIENTS

- 3 garlic cloves
- 2 bay leaves
- 3 Portobello mushrooms, cleaned, stalks removed
- 3 tbsp extra-virgin olive oil
- 6 chicken thigh fillets, trimmed
- Bunch of fresh thyme
- Juice of 2 large lemons
- 2 red chillies, deseeded and roughly chopped
- 2 avocados, halved and sliced
- Three spelt or wholemeal rolls, cut in half
- 50g rocket

METHOD

1 Mix the garlic, bay leaves and mushrooms with a tiny splash of the oil and set aside for 1 hour before seasoning and grilling at a medium heat for 10 mins each side.

2 Place chicken between 2 sheets of non-stick baking paper. Using a meat mallet (or a rolling pin), pound until 1cm thick.

3 Combine the thyme, the rest of the oil, half the lemon juice and 1 of the chillies in a bowl, season. Add the chicken and coat in mixture, cover and refrigerate for 30 mins.

4 Crush avocados with a fork, add the remaining lemon juice and chilli. Season and mix well. Remove chicken from the marinade and grill until cooked.

5 Toast the buns, then slice mushrooms on to the buns, put a handful of rocket on each, then the avocado and the chicken.

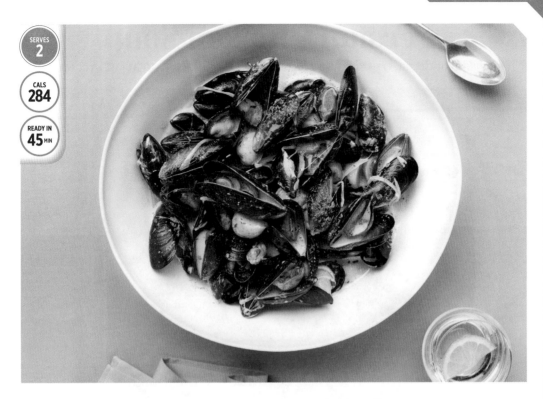

SERVES 2

CALS 284

READY IN 45 MIN

Moules Marinière

Serve up this French classic with both a skinny and a toning twist. *Formidable!*

Each portion of this fabulous French dish contains 5.8mg of zinc – 83 per cent of your RDA – which is handy, since research shows gym bunnies are more likely to be zinc deficient. Mussels are also sky-high in muscle-building protein, while the carbs in the potatoes provide energy.

INGREDIENTS
- 1kg fresh mussels
- 1 tbsp of unsalted butter
- 4 shallots, peeled and finely chopped
- 200ml of dry white wine
- Sprig of thyme
- 20g olive oil
- A pinch of curry powder
- 2 to 4 rounded tsp crème fraîche or sour cream
- 2 egg yolks
- 250g baby potatoes

METHOD

1 First, clean the mussels. Pull away the hair-like strands around the shell, yanking towards the hinge end of the mussel, then scrub them with a stiff brush in cold water. Next, cook the baby potatoes in boiling water and slice them when cooked.

2 Pour oil into a large saucepan, then add the shallots and the thyme. Stew them for 2 mins and then add mussels, dry white wine, crème fraîche and curry powder.

3 Cover the saucepan with a lid, gently shake the pan and cook over a high heat for 2-3 mins, until the mussels open.

4 Now strain the mussels into a separate pan, retaining the sauce. Time to add the egg yolks to the sauce. You can mix it with either a blender or a whisk. Lastly, add the butter, potatoes and then the mussels and pepper to the sauce.

Persian Chicken Soup

Filling and low in fat, try this twist on soup that you can whip up in just over an hour

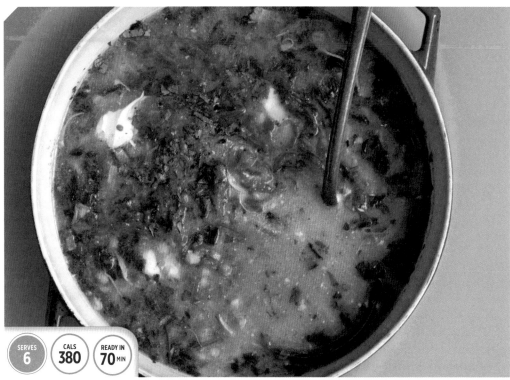

SERVES 6

CALS 380

READY IN 70 MIN

C how down on this before a big night out. The iron from the lentils, spinach and herbs will keep your energies going well into the evening, and the garlic and turmeric will support your liver in advance – think of it as a pretox. Thanks to the barley, which is high in fibre, this tasty stew will slow down the absorbtion of alcohol and protect your precious blood sugar levels. Party time.

INGREDIENTS

- 3 tsp olive oil
- 4 free-range chicken thighs or legs on the bone
- 2 large onions, chopped
- 3 garlic cloves, chopped
- 1 tsp turmeric
- 175g barley
- 75g green lentils
- Sea salt
- Black pepper
- 2 litres water
- 600ml chicken stock
- 1 small bunch of parsley
- 1 small bunch of fresh coriander
- 50g fresh spinach leaves
- 2 tbsp liquid whey or 3 tbsp 0% fat Greek yoghurt
- Zest and juice of 1 lemon

METHOD

1 Heat half the oil in a large cooking pot over a medium/high heat. Add the chicken and brown all over, then remove from the pan and set aside.

2 Add the rest of the oil and onions and sauté for 10 mins. Add the garlic and turmeric and fry for 1 min, then add the chicken, barley and lentils and season.

3 Cook for a few minutes, stirring, then add the water and stock and bring to the boil. Reduce the heat to low, cover and leave to simmer, stirring occasionally, for 45 mins.

4 Remove the chicken from the pot and shred the meat from the bone. Return the shredded meat to the pot with the fresh herbs, spinach and the liquid whey or yoghurt and bring back to the boil. Stir in the lemon juice and zest, then season with salt and pepper and ladle into bowls.

SERVES
4

CALS
174

READY IN
40 MIN

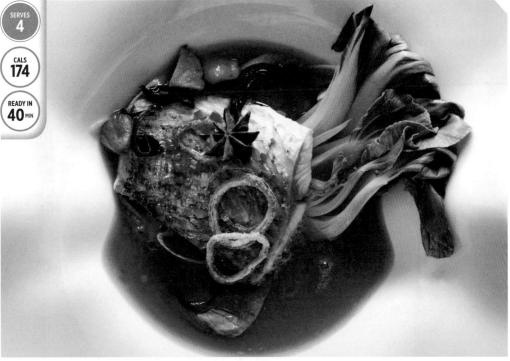

Oriental Sea Bream Broth

Impress your guests and look your best by serving this Thai-style fish dish for dinner

In an Icelandic study, subjects who ate a fish-rich diet lost, on average, 2.2lb more per month than those who didn't. Also, Scottish research suggests ginger also aids weight loss, while lemongrass gets your digestion on the move. We're hooked!

INGREDIENTS
- *4 x 500g sea bream, scaled, filleted and de-boned*
- *750ml chicken stock*
- *55ml light soy sauce*
- *50ml Thai fish sauce*
- *100g fresh ginger*
- *10 sticks fresh lemongrass, chopped*
- *1 bunch fresh coriander, finely chopped*
- *1 red chilli*
- *1 lime*
- *2 heads bok choi, cut in half*
- *400g of mixed mushrooms, chopped*
- *1 bunch of spring onions, finely chopped*

METHOD

1 First off, pour your chicken stock into a big saucepan and bring it to the boil. Then lower the heat and add the soy sauce, fish sauce, ginger, lemongrass and chilli. Leave it all to simmer for about 10 mins and then set the pan aside and allow the flavours to infuse into the liquid for 30 mins. Now pass your soup mix through a sieve to leave you with a clear broth.

2 Return the pan to a high heat and bring it back to the boil before throwing in the fish, pak choi and mushrooms. Leave the whole lot to simmer for about 5 mins.

3 Add a dash of lime to your broth, season to taste, and sprinkle on the fresh coriander leaves and spring onions to garnish. You can say *arigato* to us later.

Slow-Cooked Curry

Good things come to those who wait... Have a little patience with this low-cal cracker

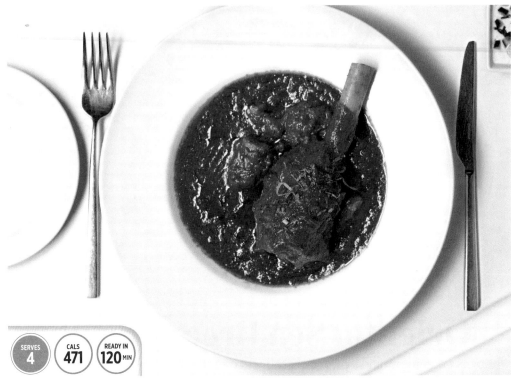

SERVES 4 · **CALS** 471 · **READY IN** 120 MIN

This tomato-based curry is lower calorie than your typical oil-slick versions (which pack around 1,000 calories), plus it's full of vitamin C, which your kidneys need to break down fats. Don't worry about the fat in the curry either – most of it is the good monounsaturated kind from the nuts.

INGREDIENTS
- 600g chicken breast, cut into chunks
- 600g sliced onion
- 300g tomatoes, sliced
- 2 tbsp of oil
- 50g cashew nuts
- 15g red chilli powder
- 10g garam masala powder
- 10g coriander powder
- 6g turmeric powder
- 3g saffron (crushed)
- 350ml chicken stock
- 10g of ginger and garlic paste
- 50g coriander leaves, chopped
- Salt to taste

METHOD

1 Mix a little of the red chilli and turmeric powder and salt. Then dip your chicken chunks into the mix until all the flesh is coated. Leave to sit for an hour while you get on with the next bit...

2 Sauté your sliced onion until it turns golden and then add the cashew nuts and ginger and garlic paste. Cook over a gentle flame for 2 mins.

3 Next, add the sliced tomato and the rest of the coriander powder, red chilli powder and turmeric powder. Leave it to cook for 30 mins. Once cooled, give the mix a whizz in the blender to make a puree.

4 Heat the oil over a low flame, then add the chicken, sauce and stock. Cook until the meat is tender. Finish the gravy with the garam masala and crushed saffron powder. Serve garnished with coriander leaves.

* BOMBAYBRASSERIELONDON.COM · QUILON.CO.UK · NUTRITIONAL INFORMATION: PRIYA TEW, DIETITIANUK.CO.UK

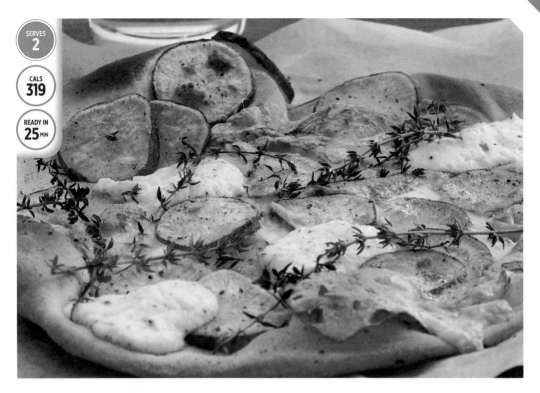

SERVES
2

CALS
319

READY IN
25 MIN

Sweet Potato & Taleggio Pizza

Step away from the pepperoni and try this tasty alternative. Easy cheesy

A healthy (but no less tasty) topping for your pizza, sweet potatoes rule the roost when it comes to flat belly benefits. As well as sporting an impressively low GI compared to white potatoes, they're full of glutathione, an antioxidant that enhances your body's metabolism. Result!

INGREDIENTS
- 3 sweet potatoes, thinly sliced
- 1 tbsp olive oil
- 2 prepared pizza bases
- 2 slices Taleggio cheese
- 3 tbsp crème fraîche
- 1 sprig of fresh thyme

METHOD

1 Preheat your oven to 220°C. Now add the sweet potato slices to a pan of salted water, bring to the boil, then simmer for 5 mins until they soften without losing shape.

2 Drain the slices and lay them on kitchen paper to blot up the excess water, then toss lightly in the olive oil and place on the pizza bases. Top the stack with shreds of the Taleggio, blobs of crème fraîche and fresh thyme. Now head to the oven.

3 Bake for about 20 mins or until the bases are crisp, the cheese golden, the herbs fra grant and your mouth drooling.

Chicken Tagine

Look no further than this warming dish for flat belly comfort food

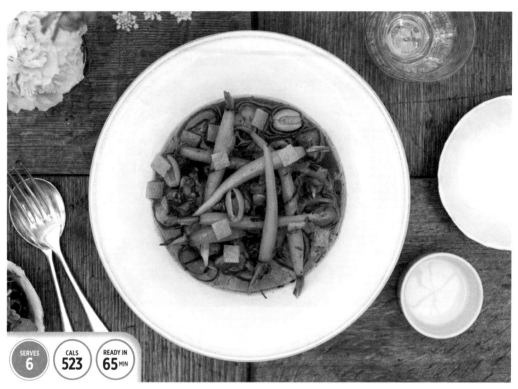

SERVES 6 | **CALS** 523 | **READY IN** 65 MIN

Chillis are packed with capsaicin, which research shows can raise your metabolism for up to five hours after you eat it. Now that is hot. Also, the lean protein in chicken breast keeps blood sugar levels constant and reduces cravings.

INGREDIENTS

- 1 tsp ground cumin
- 1 tsp ground ginger
- 1 tsp ground coriander
- 3 tsp Turkish chilli or red chilli powder
- 15 saffron threads
- 2 tbsp oil
- 2 garlic cloves, crushed with 1 tsp sea salt
- 1.4kg chicken skinless breast cut into chunks
- 400g brown onions
- 2 bunches baby carrots,
- 1 whole preserved lemon
- 800ml chicken stock
- 10 large green olives
- 50ml lemon juice
- 20g flat-leaf parsley
- 20g coriander

METHOD

1. Place the garlic, cumin, ginger, ground coriander, Turkish chilli, saffron threads and half the oil in a large bowl. Mix together, then coat the chicken in the marinade.

2. Next, tip the rest of the oil into a stainless steel pan on medium heat. Add the onions and sauté for 5-7 mins or until softened. Pop in a bowl.

3. Tip the chicken pieces into the hot pan and sauté for 5-7 mins or until golden brown, then add the carrots. Pop in the onions and cover it all with the stock.

4. Bring to the boil and then simmer over a low heat for 20-30 mins. Stir in the preserved lemon, lemon juice and olives and simmer for another 15 mins or until the sauce thickens. Serve with the herb garnish and tuck in.

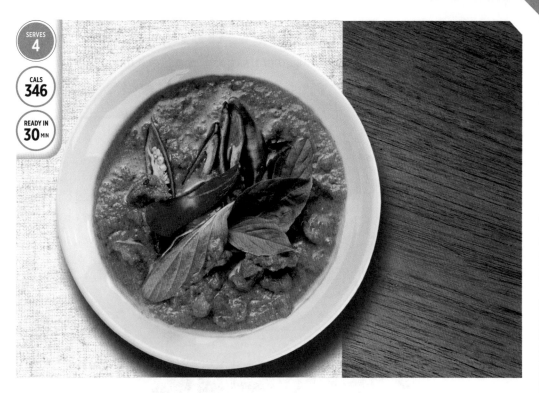

SERVES
4

CALS
346

READY IN
30 MIN

Andhra Curry

Good for your figure and your finances, this meal uses leftovers and a lot of flavour

This spicy dish from celebrity chef Anjum Anand turns a classic British roast into an exotic Indian curry – handy if you've got leftovers, but also great as a timesaver if you buy ready-cooked. The wealth of antioxidants in the chilli, ginger and spices will keep your metabolism running at full blast, while the cumin in particular will support digestion. The recipe for flat belly perfection.

INGREDIENTS
- 400g roast beef
- 20g ginger, peeled
- 2 tbsp vegetable oil
- 2 tbsp low-fat yoghurt
- 2 tsp coriander powder
- 2 tsp fennel seeds
- ½ tsp red chilli powder
- ½ tsp cumin powder
- ½ tsp turmeric powder
- 1 medium onion
- 6 cloves garlic, peeled
- 2 tomatoes, blended to a smooth purée
- 14 fresh curry leaves
- 4 dried red chillis
- ½ inch cinnamon shard

METHOD

1 Grind the cloves, cinnamon, dried chillis and fennel seeds to a fine powder. Then blend the ginger and garlic with a few drops of water to create a paste.

2 Next, throw some of the oil into a medium non-stick pan and sauté the onions. Stir in the ginger and garlic paste, cook until all the water evaporates, then add the tomatoes, yoghurt and curry leaves. Stir over a high heat for 6-8 mins.

3 Add the powdered spices, salt and a splash of water. Cook until the pan dries. Add a bit more water and cook on a medium flame until it has reduced again.

4 Finally, add 150ml water and bring to the boil. Add the beef and simmer for 4-5 mins. Then just season to taste. Now sit back with that box set.

Poussin Curry

Feel like a spring chicken? Throw together this quick curry for a mood-lifting meal

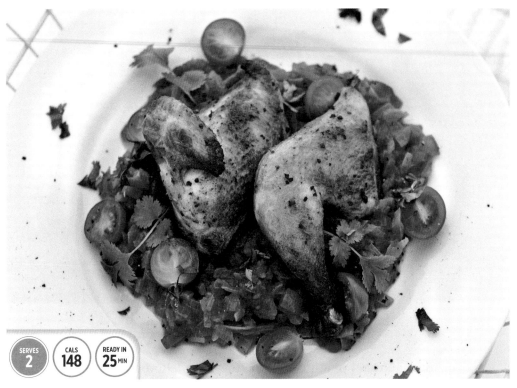

SERVES **2**   CALS **148**   READY IN **25** MIN

Just got back from the gym? This combination of tender poussin and fiery garlic and ginger is a great tonic for sore muscles. Coming from younger birds, poussin is an extra-tender form of chicken – but you can just as easily use the everyday option in this tasty dish. No fowl play here.

INGREDIENTS

- 1 poussin, cut into pieces
- 2 onions, chopped
- 5 cherry tomatoes, halved
- 1 tbsp finely chopped coriander
- 1 tsp olive oil
- ½ tbsp garlic and ginger paste
- ½ tsp garam masala
- ½ tsp chilli powder
- ½ tsp ground cumin
- 1 tsp ground coriander
- ½ tsp curry powder

METHOD

1 Start by heating the oil in a non-stick pan over a high heat and fry the poussin until browned. Remove and set aside, but keep hold of the fat – it's about to come in handy.

2 Next, heat 3 tbsp of the fat in another pan and sauté the onions. Add the paste, cook for 2–3 mins, add the garam masala, salt, a drop of water and cook for 3-4 mins.

3 Add the spices and stir. Pour in 750ml water. Add the poussin, then bring to the boil and cook on a low heat until the sauce has thickened. Add the tomatoes and coriander a few minutes from the end. Serve the sauce with the poussin on top; garnish with coriander and tuck in.

ADDITIONAL WORDS: FREYA CARR NUTRITIONAL INFORMATION: VICKI EDGSON (VICKIEDGSON.COM). PRICES CORRECT AT TIME OF GOING TO PRESS

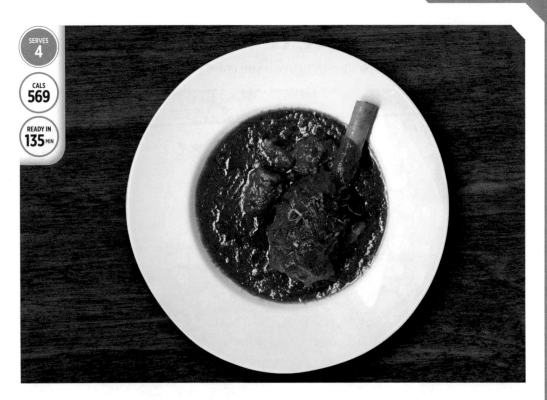

Lamb Shank

Go nuts for this meaty dinner that packs a protein punch

Nuts, particularly cashews, are great for gym bunnies, since they're high in protein and monounsaturated fatty acids – needed for energy and to absorb fat-soluble nutrients. They're also a great source of magnesium, which is essential for building muscle tissue. Impressive stuff.

INGREDIENTS

- 4 lamb shanks
- 1kg sliced onion
- 300g tomatoes, sliced
- 2 tbsp oil
- 100g cashew nuts
- 25g red chilli powder
- 10g garam masala powder
- 20g coriander powder
- 10g turmeric powder
- 3g saffron (crushed)
- 500 ml lamb stock
- 15g of ginger and garlic paste

METHOD

1 Mix a little red chilli powder, turmeric powder and salt. Dunk lamb shanks in the spice mix so that they are fully coated. Leave for an hour.

2 Meanwhile, sauté the onions in the oil. Add the cashew nuts, ginger and garlic paste. Cook over a low flame for 2 mins.

3 Add the sliced tomato and the coriander, red chilli and turmeric powders. Leave it all to bubble away for 30 mins, then pop it in the blender until you have a puree.

4 Sear the lamb shanks over a low flame and add the sauce and lamb stock. Simmer until the shanks become tender.

5 Finish your gravy with garam masala and crushed saffron powder. Serve the lamb shanks on warm plates and pour the gravy over the top.

Courgette & Mint Pizza

Another ingenious topping alternative if you crave pizza but seek the flat belly

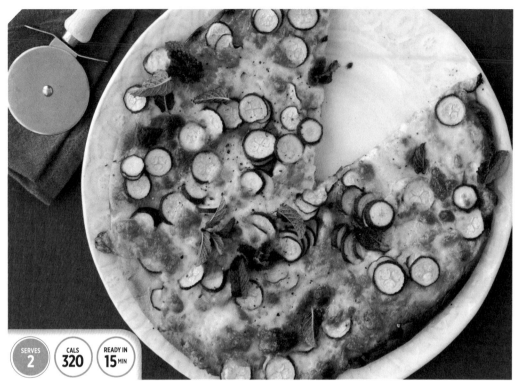

SERVES 2 · **CALS** 320 · **READY IN** 15 MIN

The courgettes in this low-calorie beauty are loaded with vitamin C, which will support your body's ability to burn fat. Plus, the mint will keep your digestion system running like a Maserati engine. Petrol not included.

INGREDIENTS
- 2 pizza bases
- 100g mozzarella, grated
- 5 medium-sized courgettes, thinly sliced into rounds
- 1 generous handful of fresh mint

METHOD

1 Fire up the oven to 220°C. Right, got the pizza bases ready and your courgettes and cheese sliced? This isn't going to take long.

2 Top each base with half the cheese and courgettes. Easy does it. Now put your feet up for 15 mins while it bakes and bubbles to golden perfection.

3 All done. Place the pizzas on a swanky wooden platter and season. Now tear up the mint and scatter on top. All done – how refreshingly simple.

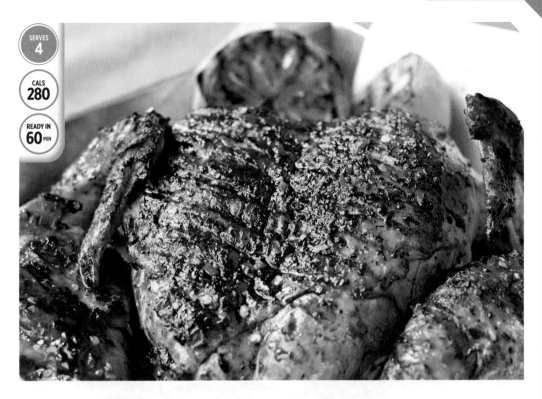

SERVES
4

CALS
280

READY IN
60 MIN

Chicken Under a Brick

Much less violent than it sounds, this Italian method will have you clucking with joy

This summer when you gather friends round for a barbecue forget smothering your food in sugar-loaded sauce. The Italians have a magic way to cook chicken that involves no special glazes, just a brick or two, some tin foil, some chilli and a couple of lemons – pair this with a salad and you've escaped the fat-laden burger stack in sophisticated style. Garden parties just got waaaaaay easier.

INGREDIENTS

- A good glug of olive oil
- 3 lemons, one juiced and zested, the others halved
- 1 tsp chilli flakes
- 1 tsp salt
- ½ tsp black pepper
- 1 whole chicken back removed and split in two (ask your butcher to do this for you)
- 2 bricks covered in aluminium foil

METHOD

1 Light the barbecue. Combine the olive oil, lemon zest and juice, chilli flakes, salt and pepper in a large bowl. Now add the chicken and give a few turns to coat. Cover and marinate in the fridge for at least 30 mins and up to 4 hours.

2 Once the flames have died down, take the chicken from the marinade and place it on the grill, skin side up. After 10 mins flip the chicken over and place a brick on top of each half. Cook for 15-20 mins until the skin is thoroughly browned and crisp and the meat pulls away easily from the bone. While the chicken cooks, toss the lemon halves on the grill for a few minutes.

3 Separate each breast from the chicken leg by making a cut right at the side bone. Serve each of the four pieces of chicken with a grilled lemon half. *Bellissimo.*

Thai Prawn Broth

Eat up and slim down with this oriental-inspired prawn and noodle dish

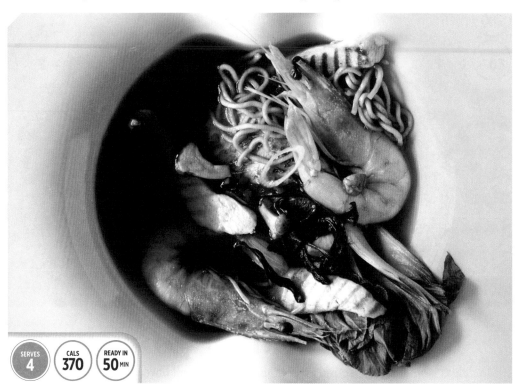

SERVES **4** CALS **370** READY IN **50** MIN

Why is this meal so good for you, you ask? Well, prawns are packed with protein and omega-3, both vital to build lean muscle, while rice noodles are the perfect post-workout carbs. Each serving has just 20mg of sodium, compared to 790mg in ramen noodles. The result: no bloating. Bliss.

INGREDIENTS

- 4 x 500g sea bream, scaled, filleted and de-boned
- 750ml chicken stock
- 55ml light soy sauce
- 50ml Thai fish sauce
- 100g fresh ginger
- 10 sticks fresh lemongrass
- 1 bunch fresh coriander
- 1 red chilli
- 1 lime
- 2 heads of bok choi
- 400g of mixed mushrooms, chopped
- 1 bunch of spring onions, finely chopped
- 250g chicken fillets
- 100g cooked prawns
- 250g rice noodles

METHOD

1 Dice the chicken fillets and pan fry them in a dash of olive oil over a medium heat for 6-8 mins. Then set it aside while you get down to making your broth.

2 Pour your chicken stock into a big pan and bring it to the boil. Add the soy sauce, fish sauce, ginger, lemon grass and chilli and simmer for 10 mins. Then take the pan off the heat and leave to infuse for 30 mins. Sieve the lot to leave you with a clear broth.

3 Bring the broth back to the boil and add the fish, cooked chicken, prawns and noodles, plus the mushrooms and bok choi, then simmer for 5 mins or so.

4 Now just add a dash of lime, season and garnish with the fresh coriander and spring onion. Grab your biggest soup spoon – and start slurping.

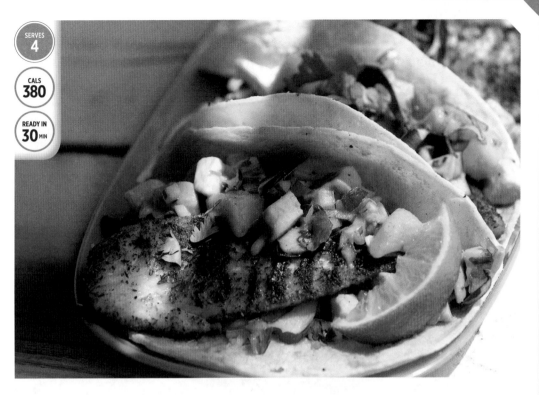

SERVES
4

CALS
380

READY IN
30 MIN

Grilled Fish Tacos

Avoid the added mayo at the Mexican by trying these tacos at home

Order these in a restaurant or grab a pre-made supermarket version and you'll find the fish gets a good battering and a massive dollop of mayonnaise before it reaches your table. So we ditched the frying oil and fatty dressing but kept the flavour by using a spicy Cajun seasoning and a nutrient-rich mango and avocado salsa, which cuts the heat and pairs perfectly with the fish.

INGREDIENTS
- 1 mango, peeled, pitted and cubed
- 1 avocado, peeled, pitted and cubed
- ½ red onion, finely chopped
- Juice of 1 lime / wedges to garnish
- Chopped fresh coriander
- A splash of canola oil
- 2 large swordfish fillets
- 1 tbsp Cajun seasoning
- 8 corn tortillas
- 2 handfuls shredded red cabbage

METHOD

1 Mix the mango, avocado, onion and lime juice in a bowl to make the salsa. Season to taste salt and pepper and add coriander.

2 Heat a grill or griddle pan until hot. Drizzle a light coating of oil over the fish and rub on the Cajun spice. Cook the fish, undisturbed, for 4 mins. Flip with a spatula – careful now – and cook for another 4 mins, then remove to a plate.

3 Warm the tortillas on the grill for a minute or two, or if you're in the kitchen wrap in damp paper towels and microwave for 1 min until warm and pliable.

4 Break the fish into chunks and divide among the warm tortillas. Top with the cabbage and the mango salsa. Serve with the lime wedges. Heaven.

Sweet Pistachio Chicken

Go nuts for this pistachio dish – as good for your taste buds as it is for your waistline

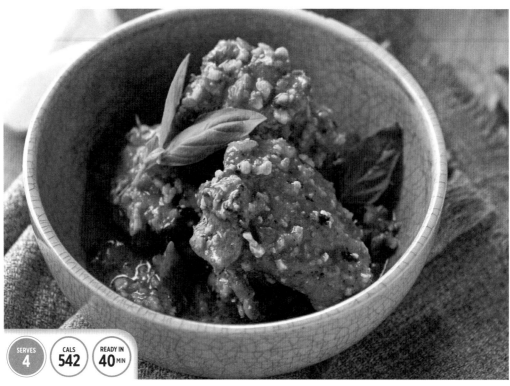

SERVES 4 · **CALS** 542 · **READY IN** 40 MIN

Ahhh, where would our flat bellies be without the classic, muscle-pleasing meat and nut protein combo? Here's a fragrant twist on the magic formula, with added antioxidant-loaded thyme and garlic. Pistachios are jam-packed with vitamin B6, which helps your body break down protein and use it as effectively as possible. Nutty, but true.

INGREDIENTS

- 60ml extra-virgin olive oil
- 1 tbsp thyme leaves
- Salt and freshly ground black pepper, to taste
- 4 chicken breast fillets
- 2 garlic cloves, sliced
- 80ml apple cider vinegar
- 2 tbsp rice malt syrup
- 6 drops stevia liquid
- 125ml chicken stock
- 65g chopped pistachios

METHOD

1 Mix 1 tbsp of the olive oil, then the thyme, salt and pepper in a bowl. Rub the marinade into the chicken.

2 Heat 1 tbsp of the oil in a heavy-based frying pan over a medium heat and sauté the garlic for 5 mins. Add the chicken and cook for 15 to 20 mins, turning regularly.

3 Remove the chicken from the pan, set aside in a serving dish and keep warm. Then put the vinegar, rice malt syrup and remaining oil in a saucepan and cook for 1 min, stirring constantly.

4 Add the stevia and stock to the pan and simmer for about 10 mins, until it thickens. Add the pistachios, then pour sauce over the chicken and serve. Dig in.

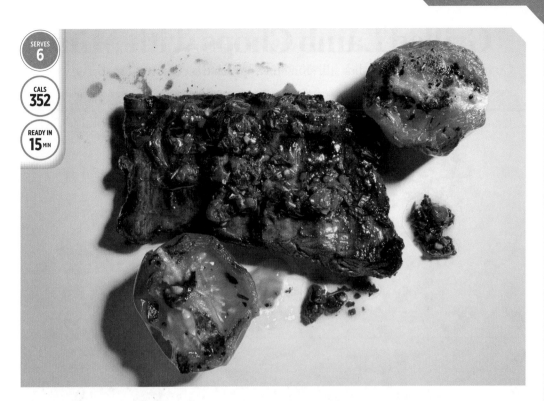

SERVES
6

CALS
352

READY IN
15 MIN

Skirt Steak with Chimichurri

There's nothing girly about this meaty meal. Get stuck in for a serious health kick

A traditional Argentine sauce, chimichurri is a damn sight better for you than ketchup. With not one, not two, but nine cloves of garlic in total (now that's a kick up the backside for your metabolism), as well as vitamin K-packed and antioxidant-rich oregano, this recipe will get your fires burning. Just don't blame us if no one wants to kiss you after, okay?

INGREDIENTS

- 9 cloves garlic, finely chopped
- 1 bunch parsley, chopped
- 1 bunch oregano, chopped
- ½ bunch spring onions, chopped
- 1 tsp paprika
- Juice of 2 lemons
- 60ml balsamic vinegar
- 150ml olive oil
- 3 x 400g skirt steaks
- 6 plum tomatoes
- 1 tsp olive oil

METHOD

1 Make the chimichurri. Mix two-thirds of the garlic, the herbs, spring onions, paprika, lemon juice and balsamic, leave for 1 hour, then whisk in the oil and season. It's ideal to do this at least two days before you need it, to allow the flavour to form.

2 Put your tomatoes in half and mix them with the rest of the garlic, salt, pepper and enough olive oil to coat. Rest overnight.

3 Get the grill ready and make sure the steaks are at room temperature – and don't season them before cooking. Grill the tomatoes at a lower heat on the outside of the grill, until you get char marks. Cook the steaks on the hottest part of the grill for 4 mins per side, then rest for them for 5 mins.

4 Slice the steaks, transfer to a big platter together with your grilled tomatoes and drizzle with the chimichurri. Get stuck in.

Grilled Lamb Chops with Mint

You can meat up – but still slim down – with this Argentine barbecue

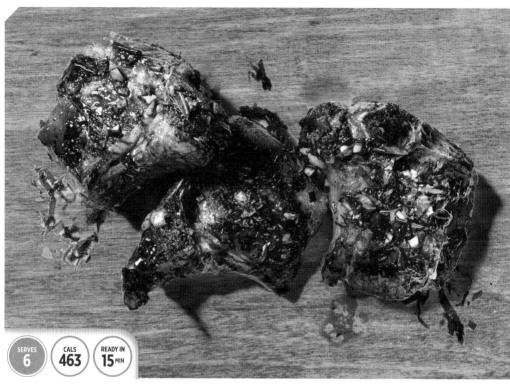

SERVES 6 · **CALS** 463 · **READY IN** 15 MIN

According to the Wheeling Jesuit University, the scent of peppermint alone can act as an appetite suppressant, so teaming it with meat can stop overindulgence. That might explain why Argentines stay so healthy despite a diet that's heavy in red meat – they put mint with everything! This recipe is best barbecued, but an oven grill can work too.

INGREDIENTS

- 12 lamb chops
- 1 tbsp rosemary
- 3 large cloves garlic, crushed
- 1 tbsp thyme leaves
- 1 tsp cayenne pepper
- 1 tsp cumin
- 5 tbsp extra-virgin olive oil
- 100g chopped anchovies
- 1 bunch fresh mint, chopped

METHOD

1 Get the grill on! Marinate the lamb chops in a bowl with the rosemary, garlic, thyme, cayenne pepper, cumin and 3 tbsp of the oil, all mixed well. Leave for at least 1 hour.

2 Remove the chops from the marinade – put this to one side – and grill at a fierce heat for 3 mins on each side, adding sea salt at each turn. You want to get a nice crust on the outside and pink all way through.

3 Once done, move the lamb chops to a less hot area of the grill for 7 more mins.

4 Now gently heat the marinade in a small pan with the rest of the olive oil, the anchovies and mint. When done, arrange the lamb chops on a big platter topped with the warm marinade and sprinkled with more chopped mint.

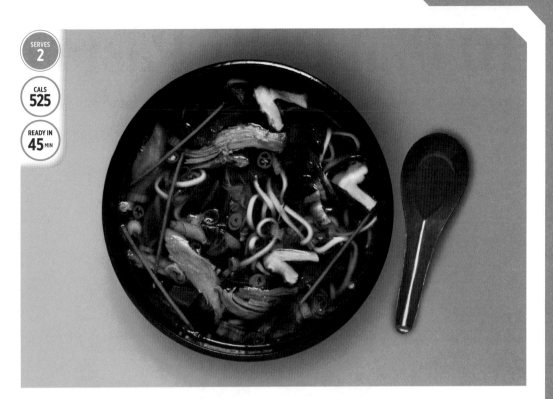

SERVES
2

CALS
525

READY IN
45 MIN

Roast Duck Noodle Soup

Get quacking with this warming, protein-packed dish – perfect for after the gym

You'd be forgiven for thinking that duck is off the menu for flat belly folk, but it's a great source of protein and rich in vitamin B3 and iron, which both are vital to an efficient metabolism. Pair this with the chilli, ginger, and garlic and you're looking at some mighty fat-burning power. Also, ginger is stacked with anti-inflammatory compounds that can help soothe sore post-gym muscles. That's better.

INGREDIENTS
- 250g duck leg
- 1 tbsp honey
- 1 tsp Chinese five-spice
- 1 tbsp soy sauce
- 100g egg noodles
- 1 litre chicken stock
- 1 inch ginger,
- 1 garlic clove, bashed
- 1 star anise
- 2 tbsp oyster sauce
- 1 tsp sesame oil
- 3 shiitake mushrooms
- 2 heads of bok choi, sliced
- 50g enoki mushrooms
- 4 spring onions, sliced
- A few chives, sliced
- 1 red bird's eye chilli
- A few fresh mint leaves

METHOD

1 Heat the oven to 180°C. Rub the duck leg with salt and pepper. Roast it for 45 mins, until the skin is crispy and the meat tender.

2 Mix together honey, five-spice and half of the soy sauce in a large pan. Place the duck leg in it and put over a medium heat. Cook gently until sticky and glossy. Remove the leg from the pan and shred the meat.

3 Cook the noodles in a saucepan of boiling water with a pinch of salt until tender. Drain. Heat the stock, ginger, garlic and star anise in a large pan, add the oyster sauce, sesame oil and remaining soy sauce.

4 Discard the ginger, garlic and star anise. Add the shiitakes and cook for 3 mins, then add bok choi, enoki, spring onions, chives, noodles and duck. Boil, then remove from heat. Serve in bowls garnished with the chopped chilli and mint. Dig in.

10 Flat Belly Pastas

Michelin-starred chef Angela Hartnett plates up 10 genius sauces that will fire up your metabolism and fight fat. *Pasta la vista*

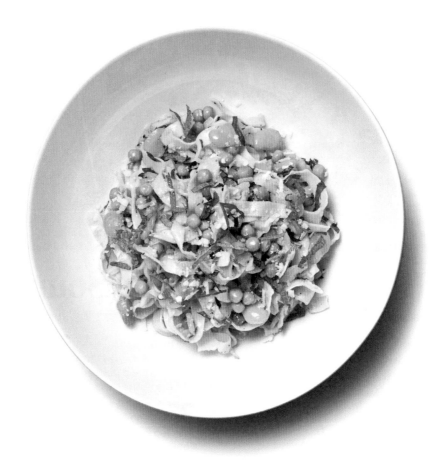

1: TUMMY-FILLING PEA TAGLIATELLE
SERVES 4 | CALS 538 | READY IN 15 MINS

200g fresh peas • 200g fresh broad beans • 1 garlic clove, crushed • 50ml olive oil • 600g fresh tagliatelle • Handful mint, chopped • 50g Parmesan, grated

Mama mia! Not only is this dish delish, you can make it in just 15 mins. Cook the peas and beans in salted water for 2-3 mins. Drain and plunge into iced water. Cook the garlic in oil for 1 min, then add the drained peas and beans for a further 2 mins. Remove from the heat. Cook the tagliatelle until *al dente*, drain and add to the pea mix. Toss, season and add chopped mint. Serve with Parmesan. This serving of broad beans and peas has 22 per cent of your RDA of fibre, essential if you want to lose weight.

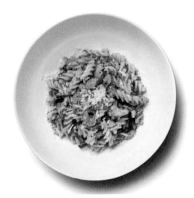

2: FILLING PANCETTA FUSILLI
SERVES 4 | CALS 760 | READY IN 20 MINS

1 cauliflower • 375g dried fusilli • 1 tbsp olive oil • 100g pancetta, chopped • 100g pine nuts • 100g raisins • 2 tbsp chopped flat leaf parsley • Grated Parmesan, to serve

Pine nuts might be tiny but they scare off the munchies. Boil cauliflower until soft. Remove, but keep the water and bring it back to the boil to cook the pasta. Sauté the pancetta in a pan. Add cauliflower, nuts and raisins and season. Drain pasta and mix in, with parsley and Parmesan.

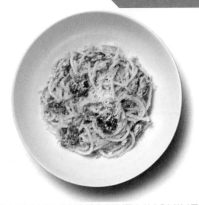

3: HEALTHY WALNUT LINGUINE
SERVES 4 | CALS 879 | READY IN 10 MINS

200g walnuts • 2 tbsp breadcrumbs • 25g butter • 100ml crème fraîche • 375g dried linguine • 50g Parmesan, grated • 1 tbsp chopped flat leaf parsley

Soften walnuts in boiling water, then crush to a purée in a bowl. Add breadcrumbs and butter, add crème fraîche and season. Cook pasta. Drain, put back in the pan with the walnut mix. Finish with Parmesan and parsley, and let the walnuts' omega-3 do its fat-busting work.

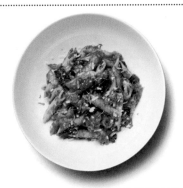

4: SLOW-BURN AUBERGINE RIGATONI
SERVES 4 | CALS 464 | READY IN 50 MINS

1 aubergine • 2 tbsp olive oil • 2 garlic cloves, crushed • 100ml red wine vinegar • 6 tomatoes, diced • 375g dried rigatoni • 125g ricotta salata, grated • Handful basil

Weight loss demands fibre, and aubergine has it in droves. Slice aubergine into 5 x 2.5cm strips. Place in a colander, sprinkle with salt, and drain for 30 mins. Sauté the garlic and aubergine until golden. Add the vinegar, then tomatoes and cook for 10 mins. Cook pasta, add the ricotta and basil.

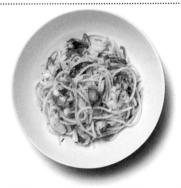

5: TONE-UP LOBSTER LINGUINE
SERVES 4 | CALS 635 | READY IN 20 MINS

2 cooked lobsters • 320g dried linguine • 2 tbsp olive oil • 1 garlic clove, crushed • 4 spring onions, finely chopped • ½ tsp finely chopped red chilli • 25ml dry white wine • 1 tbsp chopped flat leaf parsley

Cut lobster meat into bite-size pieces and cook the pasta. Heat the oil in a pan, add the garlic, onions and chilli and fry for 1 min. Stir in the lobster and heat for 1 min. Add the wine and reduce. Drain the linguine and add to the pan. Stir in the parsley and season.

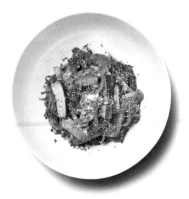

6: NO-CARB COURGETTE PENNE
SERVES 4 | CALS 233 | READY IN 40 MINS

4 courgettes • 4 tbsp olive oil • 1 onion, chopped • 800g plum tomatoes • 1 garlic clove, chopped • 2 tsp tomato purée • Pinch sugar • 1 sprig rosemary

Cut courgettes into penne shapes and blanch in boiling water for 2-3 mins. Heat the oil and cook the onion. Squash tomatoes with a fork and add to the pan with garlic, purée, sugar and rosemary. Simmer for 30 mins. Remove rosemary, mix with courgette and drizzle with olive oil.

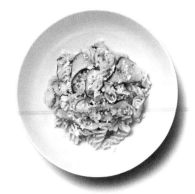

7: FAT-FIGHTING COURGETTE FUSILLI
SERVES 4 | CALS 497 | READY IN 10 MINS

375g dried fusilli • 2 courgettes • 4 tbsp olive oil • 1 tsp chopped chilli • 2 garlic cloves, finely sliced • Handful grated pecorino cheese

Cook pasta. While it's boiling, cut the courgette lengthways into thin strips. Heat 2 tbsp oil and sauté the chilli, garlic and courgette for 3 mins, without colouring. Season and set aside. Drain pasta and toss with the courgette mix. Finish with pecorino and the rest of the oil.

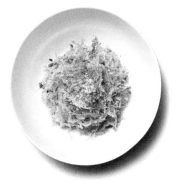

8: METABOLIC SPAGHETTI SQUASH
SERVES 4 | CALS 588 | READY IN 35 MINS

1 spaghetti squash • 2 tbsp olive oil • 1 garlic clove, sliced • 2 dried red chillies, crushed • 1 tbsp chopped flat leaf parsley • Handful grated Parmesan cheese

Another no-carb option. Cut squash in half, remove seeds and bake for 30 mins before scraping out with a fork. For the sauce, fry garlic and chillies for 30 seconds. Remove from heat and add the squash strands. Stir in parsley, season and add Parmesan. Microwave for 2 mins.

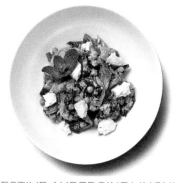

9: DIGESTIVE AUBERGINE LINGUINE
SERVES 4 | CALS 505 | READY IN 20 MINS

3 aubergines • 100ml olive oil • 200g fresh peas • 1 garlic clove, crushed • 200g crumbled goat's cheese • Handful mint, chopped • Handful grated Parmesan cheese

Cut aubergine into 1cm-wide strips, sprinkle with salt and drain for 15 mins. Rinse, then fry in 50ml oil. Cook peas for 2-3 mins. Heat the remaining oil, add garlic for 1 min, then peas for 2-3 mins. Mix with goat's cheese, aubergine and serve with mint, Parmesan and a drizzle of oil.

10: BIG VITS MUSSELS LINGUINE
SERVES 4 | CALS 770 | READY IN 25 MINS

2kg mussels • 350g linguine
• 2 tbsp olive oil • 1 garlic clove,
sliced • Pinch chilli powder
• 250g tomatoes • Zest of 1
lemon • 1 tbsp chopped parsley
• 1 tbsp torn basil

The mineral content of mussels rivals that of red meat but minus the fat, and they have just as much vitamin C as the tomatoes in this dish. Scrub the mussels, remove the beards and sit them in cold water for 10 mins. Add to a hot, dry, lidded pan and steam for 5 mins, until they open. Cool, remove shells, then cook the linguine. Heat 1 tbsp oil, add garlic, chilli and chopped tomatoes, cook for 5 mins. Drain the pasta and toss with the mussels and sauce. Serve with the rest of the oil, the zest and herbs.

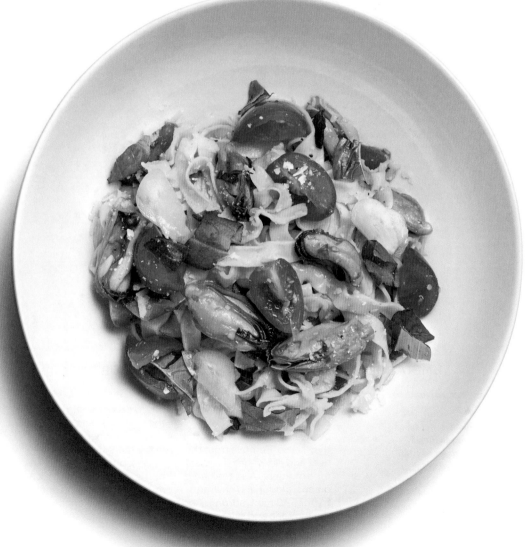

10 Slimming Spices

Gurpareet Bains, author of Indian Superspices, rustles up five body-boosting curries, plus the ultimate detox drinks to have with them

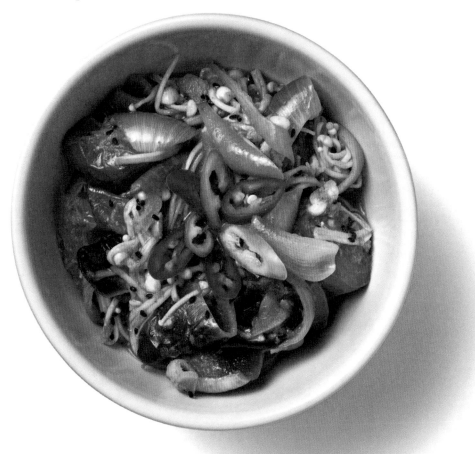

1: METABOLISM-BOOSTING OYSTER MUSHROOM SUBZI
SERVES 2-3 | CALS 150 | READY IN 30 MINS

Dash of olive oil • 1 tbsp nigella seeds • 4 garlic cloves, chopped • 2 small onions, quartered • 1 tbsp grated ginger • 1 green chilli • 1 tsp turmeric • Salt, to taste • 2 tomatoes • 250g oyster mushrooms • 100ml light coconut milk

Pour some oil into a frying pan, add seeds and cook over a low-medium heat until they sizzle. Remove from the heat and allow the oil to cool for a moment. Add the garlic, onions, ginger and chilli and fry for 5-10 mins, stirring. Add the turmeric and salt and cook for 20 seconds, stirring. Add the tomatoes and cook until soft – no longer than 5 mins. In the meantime, wipe the mushrooms clean. Once the pan is ready, add the milk and mushrooms. Stir and cook over a low heat, uncovered, for 10 mins, then serve.

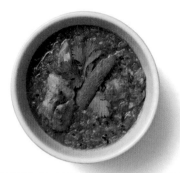

2: ANTIOXIDANT CHICKEN MADRAS
SERVES 4 | CALS 205 | READY IN 1 HR

Olive oil • 2 tbsp nigella seeds • 1 tbsp fennel seeds • 1 tbsp fenugreek seeds • 2 cinnamon sticks • 1 garlic bulb • 4 tbsp grated ginger • 1 tbsp turmeric • 1 tsp ground ginger • 2 tsp chilli powder • 2 onions • 1 tbsp tomato purée • 1 tbsp tamarind paste • 700g chicken joints, skinned • 1 tsp garam masala • 25g coriander

Fry the seeds and cinnamon in a pan for 2-3 mins. Remove from the heat, cool. Add the garlic and ginger and cook for 2-3 mins, stirring. Mix in the turmeric, ginger, chilli and salt, then add onions, purée, paste and chicken. Cook for 10 mins. Add boiling water to cover the chicken, bring to the boil, reduce to a simmer and cook for 45 mins. Add garam masala and coriander.

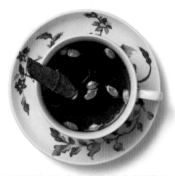

3: SOOTHING ROOIBOS TEA
MAKES 3 MUGS | CALS 0 | READY IN 12 MINS

1 organic rooibos tea bag • 2 cinnamon sticks • 5 green cardamom pods, lightly crushed • Large pinch ground ginger • Large pinch saffron • 3 tbsp runny honey

The stress hormone cortisol loves to pack on belly fat – chill out and slim down. Place the tea bag, cinnamon sticks, green cardamom pods, ground ginger, saffron and honey in a pan. Add 3 mugs cold water and bring to the boil. Reduce to a low heat, pop a lid on and simmer for 10 mins. Remove from the heat and pour the mixture into three mugs through a strainer.

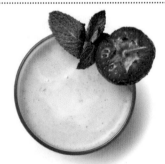

4: SLIMMING STRAWBERRY LASSI
SERVES 2-3 | CALS 60 | READY IN 2 MINS

250g strawberries • 1 tsp fennel seeds • fresh mint • 200ml yoghurt • Handful ice, plus extra • Sugar, to taste

Put all the ingredients in a blender and whizz. Place extra ice in glasses and pour in the lassi. Decorate with a mint leaf and serve. The berries here will regulate blood sugar and load you up with metabolism-boosting vitamin C, and fennel and mint both act as effective digestion aids.

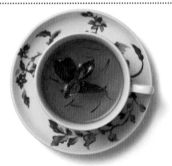

5: MINT AND SAFFRON TUMMY TEA
MAKES 2 MUGS | CALS 0 | READY IN 12 MINS

1 green tea bag • 1 tsp saffron • Fresh mint • Honey, to taste

Settle your stomach with mint, while the antioxidant saffron spring-cleans your system. Place the tea bag and saffron in a pan. Add 2 mugs of water and bring to the boil. Simmer for 10 mins. Discard the tea bag and pour into the mugs with the mint. Add honey to taste.

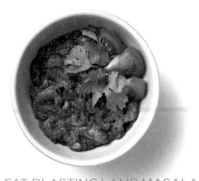

6: FAT-BLASTING LAMB MASALA
SERVES 4 | CALS 290 | READY IN 2 HRS

Olive oil • 20 cardamom pods, crushed • 1 tbsp nigella seeds • 6 cloves garlic, chopped • 4 tbsp grated ginger • 1 tsp turmeric • 1 tsp chilli powder • 1 tbsp ground nutmeg • Salt, to taste • 4 onions, diced • 2 tbsp tomato purée • 500g lean lamb leg, diced • 2 tsp garam masala • 25g coriander to season

Your liver works hard all day to burn fat – treat it to some nutmeg to say thanks. Fry pods and seeds over a medium heat for 3 mins and remove. Add garlic and ginger, cook until golden. Add chilli, turmeric, nutmeg, salt, then onions, purée and lamb, stir until the lamb is sealed. Pour in boiling water to cover the lamb and bring to the boil. Simmer and cook, uncovered, for 90 mins. Serve.

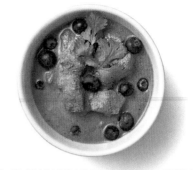

7: CLEANSING TURKEY CURRY
SERVES 4 | CALS 250 | READY IN 15 MINS

200g blueberries • 20g coriander • 4 garlic cloves • 2 tbsp grated ginger • 2 tsp ground cinnamon • 2 tsp fennel seeds • 1 tsp chilli powder • ½ tsp turmeric • 500g low-fat Greek yoghurt • 500g skinless, boneless turkey breast fillets • 1 tsp garam masala • Fresh coriander

Antioxidant soup, this. Blend the blueberries, coriander, garlic, ginger, ground cinnamon, fennel seeds, chilli powder, turmeric, salt and yoghurt to a purée. Set aside. Place the turkey in a deep saucepan and pour in the yoghurt mixture. Stir and simmer over a low heat. Cook uncovered for 10 mins before mixing through the garam masala. Garnish with more coriander and serve.

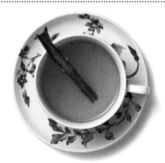

8: SLIM-DOWN SPICED TEA
MAKES 3 MUGS | CALS 0 | READY IN 12 MINS

1 green tea bag • 1 cinnamon stick • 1 tbsp fennel seeds • Pinch ground ginger

Place the tea, cinnamon, fennel seeds and ginger in a pan. Add 3 mugs of water and bring to the boil. Reduce the heat and simmer for 10 mins. Pour into mugs through a strainer. Done. Green tea can speed up the metabolism as it helps the liver function. Slurp!

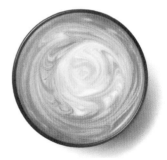

9: BODY-BOOSTING MANGO LASSI
SERVES 2-3 | CALS 94 | READY IN 5 MINS

175g diced mango • 300ml yoghurt • Pinch saffron • 1 tsp grated ginger • Handful ice, plus extra • Sugar, to taste

Another nice and easy one for you. Pop all the ingredients in a blender and whizz until you get a smooth mixture. Place the extra ice in glasses and pour over the lassi. Easy. Mango boasts a brilliant 25 antioxidants, so try this first thing for a great start to your day.

10: OMEGA-RICH SALMON GOJI CURRY

SERVES 4 | CALS 400 | READY IN 25 MINS

Olive oil • 1 tbsp nigella seeds
• 1 tbsp cumin seeds • 1 tsp
coriander seeds • 1 tsp mustard
seeds • 8 garlic cloves • 3 tbsp
grated ginger • 1 tsp turmeric
• 400g passata • Handful curry
leaves • 2 green chillies • ½ tsp
sugar • 500g salmon, skinned
and cubed • 50g goji berries
• 25g coriander

You know the drill: pour the oil into a pan, add the seeds and cook over a high heat until they pop. Allow to cool. Add the garlic and ginger and fry over a low heat until golden. Add the turmeric and cook for about 20 seconds, stirring. Add the passata, curry leaves, chillies, salt and sugar and stir. Stir in the salmon, reduce to a gentle simmer and cook, uncovered, for 4–5 mins or until the salmon is cooked, then mix in the goji berries. Top with coriander and send that protein straight to your muscles.

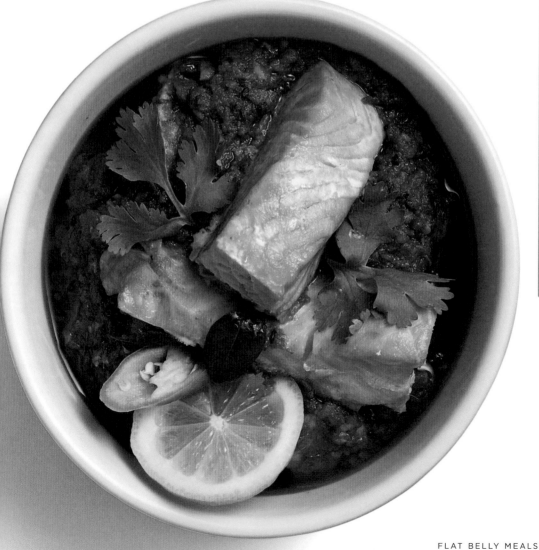

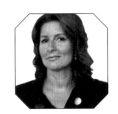

MY FLAT BELLY DIARY:

Nicky Kinnard

Space NK founder Nicky Kinnaird MBE's impressive fitness regime keeps her in fine shape. How does she fuel her flat belly schedule?

MONDAY

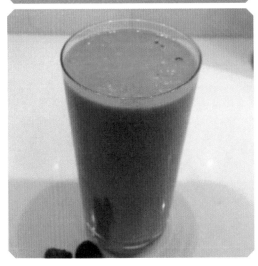

6:45am
David Kirsch Protein Plus Meal Replacement, with raspberries and a green tea

10:30am
Apple, walnuts and 1.5 litres of water

1pm
Itsu salmon and tuna sushi

8:30pm
Grilled salmon with asparagus, broccoli, beans, peas and leeks

I make sure I have a session with my trainer every Monday to go through weights and cardio routines. I end up eating late when I train after work but otherwise I make sure I eat dinner early so there's time to properly digest it all before bed.

TUESDAY

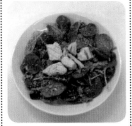

7:30am
2% Greek yoghurt with berries

12pm
Couscous salad with chicken, spinach and two glasses of water

3pm
David Kirsch Protein Plus Meal Replacement and Super Charged Greens

7:30pm
Burrata with tomatoes, basil and olive oil

I do a 5km run in the morning and always try to stay hydrated by regulating my water intake throughout the day.

WEDNESDAY

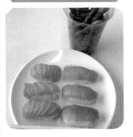

6:45am
Two boiled eggs and a green tea

11am
Banana with 1.5 litres of water

2:30pm
Itsu shrimp, tuna and salmon sushi with edamame and two glasses of water

7:30pm
Veal with peppers and beans, frozen yoghurt and two glasses of red wine

I eat out a few times a week but still try to make healthy choices. I cut back on carbs from mid-afternoon and I eat lots of green vegetables.

THURSDAY	FRIDAY	SATURDAY	SUNDAY

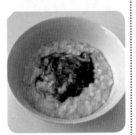 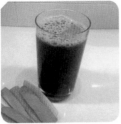 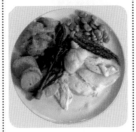 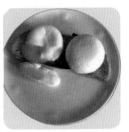

THURSDAY

7:30am
Porridge with berry compote and a green tea

1pm
Salad with fennel, peppers and cucumber, two glasses of water

3pm
Apple and raw almonds

7:30pm
Grilled salmon with asparagus, carrots, broccoli, peas and beans

I work out every day and prefer morning sessions. I go to the gym at 6-7am during the week and at weekends, I test myself with longer runs.

FRIDAY

6:45am
Cucumber, kale, celery and apple juice, with carrot and celery sticks

11am
2% Greek yoghurt with almonds and 1.5 litres of water

2pm
Tomato, broccoli and mozzarella salad

7:30pm
Steak with broccoli and two glasses of red wine

I take supplements: a daily blue/green algae one along with a multivitamin, calcium citrate, vitamin D and omega-3. Wellbeing starts from within.

SATURDAY

9:30am
David Kirsch Protein Plus Meal Replacement, with raspberries and a green tea

12pm
Skimmed latte, banana and 1.5 litres of water

3pm
2% Greek yoghurt with an apple

5:30pm
Roast chicken with green vegetables and sweet potato

I love the short, sharp bursts you get in a sweaty spin class, so I try to go at least once a week. It feels as though your legs have been well exercised.

SUNDAY

10am
Poached eggs and sourdough toast with a green tea

12:30pm
Green juice and 1.5 litres of water

2pm
2% Greek yoghurt with an apple

6pm
Roast beef with broad beans, green beans, Brussels sprouts, broccoli, carrots and cauliflower

I love running. No matter where you are, you can always bring a pair of running shoes and go out there and explore. I try to do at least 12km a week.

THE EXPERT VERDICT

Our nutritionist Dr Christy Fergusson gives her feedback: "It's obvious Nicky takes care of herself, and her diet is balanced and healthy, but there are a few small tweaks she could make.

"Nicky eats a few things you might not realise are processed. The 2% Greek yoghurt often contains the same calories – or more – than its full-fat counterpart because of sugar added to make up for the loss of taste when the fat is taken away. There's only 5g of fat per 150g pot in the full-fat variety so it isn't as naughty as you might think.

"Nicky eats a lot of salmon. Farmed salmon can be toxic, so it's important to make sure it comes from a reputable source. Swapping white rice in sushi for organic brown would have less effect on her blood-sugar levels as white rice is almost immediately converted into sugar in the body. While changing green tea to yerba mate also helps rebalance blood sugar. It's an impressive diet though."

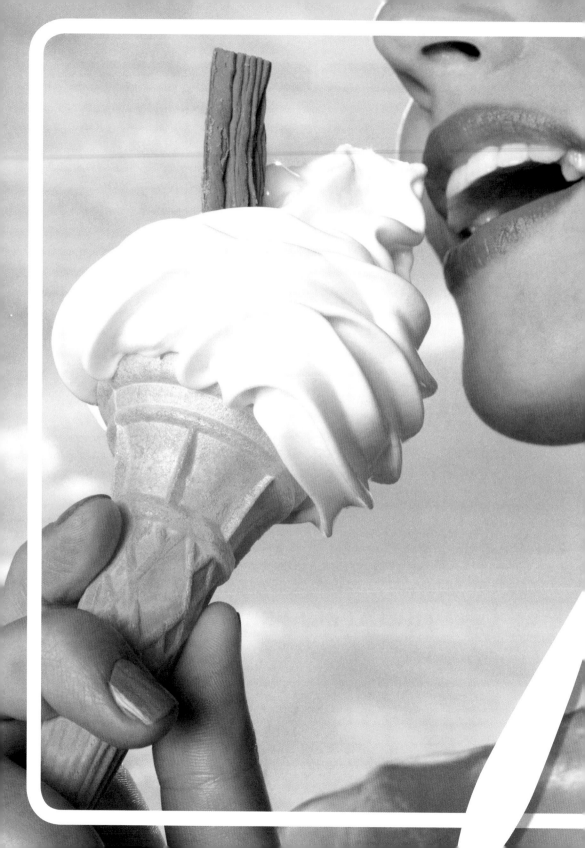

DELICIOUS DESSERTS

Life should be about balance. You could cut out desserts entirely if you want to lose weight, but that sounds less like a change in eating habits and more like a diet to us – and we all know how long those last. With just a few tweaks and clever swaps, you can enjoy these ices, puds and cakes, safe in the knowledge that they've been created with a slimmer stomach in mind.

Not So Sinful Soufflés

At 126 calories a pop, these little treats are a perfect way to indulge your sweet tooth

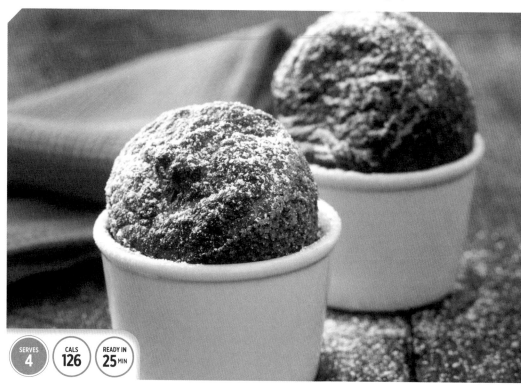

SERVES 4 **CALS** 126 **READY IN** 25 MIN

Now this is some scientific research we can really get behind: eating cocoa powder may produce an anti-inflammatory response in the body, according to new findings presented at the National Meeting & Exposition of the American Chemical Society today. Tasty!

INGREDIENTS
- 60g/2oz caster sugar
- 1 heaped tbsp cocoa powder
- 4 large egg whites
- Few drops vanilla extract
- 1 pinch cream of tartar
- 25g/1oz plain (dark) chocolate, 85% cocoa solids, roughly chopped
- Icing sugar

METHOD

1 Heat the oven to 180°C. Get ready – grease 4 ramekins or pudding basins.

2 Now sift 40g of the sugar with the cocoa into a bowl and set aside. In a Pyrex bowl, whisk the egg whites, vanilla and cream of tartar until soft peaks form. Whisk in remaining sugar until stiff.

3 Fold the sugar and cocoa mix in with the chocolate. Divide among the ramekins, wiping clean the top edges to ensure they rise evenly.

4 Put ramekins in a roasting tin filled with hot water to halfway up their sides. Cook for 10-12 mins, until risen and set around the edges.

5 Sift icing sugar on top and serve. Good, eh?

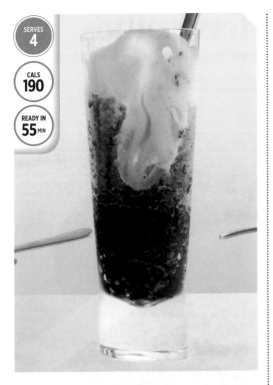

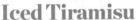

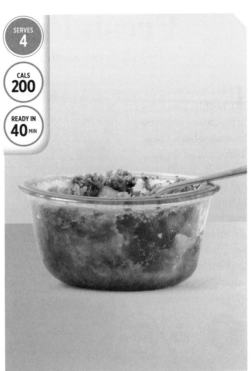

SERVES 4
CALS 190
READY IN 55 MIN

SERVES 4
CALS 200
READY IN 40 MIN

Iced Tiramisu

This clever take on a creamy tiramisu is chock-full of antioxidants and super low in calories. We've kept the indulgence of the cream, but ditched fatty sponge fingers for an espresso granita. *Bellissimo.*

50g sugar • 120ml double cream • 1 tbsp icing sugar • 2 shots hot espresso (or use instant espresso granules) • 8 chocolate-covered espresso beans, crushed (or use 2 tbsp chocolate curls instead)

1 Stir the espresso and sugar together until the sugar dissolves. Next transfer the mixture to an 8-by-8-inch baking dish and place, uncovered, in the freezer. After 45 mins, stir it with a fork to break up the ice and freeze for another 2 hours, stirring every 30 mins, until it's nice and slushy.

2 Now whip the cream with an electric mixer until soft peaks form. Add the icing sugar and beat until blended together. Next scoop the granita into four tall glasses and top with big dollops of cream and the crushed espresso beans or chocolate curls.

Slimline Crumble

It's crumble – but not as you know it. We've switched bland white flour in the topping for rolled oats and wholemeal flour, and used juicy pears with cardamom so you don't need to add a ton of sugar. Sweet!

30g rolled oats • 2 tbsp wholemeal flour • 1 tbsp brown sugar • 3 tbsp cold butter, cut into small pieces • 1 tsp ground cardamom • 1 pinch of salt • 3 ripe pears, peeled, cored and diced

1 Easiest bit first – preheat your oven to 200°C. Now pop the oats, flour, sugar and salt in your blender and pulse a few times. Add the butter and pulse the mix again until it looks clumpy (bear with us). You can do it all by hand too; it'll take longer but think of those toned biceps.

2 Next, get a big bowl out and toss the pears in it along with the cardamom. Then divide the fruit mixture into four ramekins and sprinkle on the topping until the pears are covered. Put the ramekins on a baking sheet and cook for 30 mins or until the topping is golden and crunchy.

Fresh Fruit Ice-Lollies

Not just for kids, these are sure to be a perfect fix of natural sugar for everyone

If you're looking for a healthy alternative to ice cream, forget the frozen yoghurt. These lollies will hit the spot – especially as each one has nearly a full serving of fruit in it. The type of fruit is up to you; we've got three suggestions here, but if it can go in the blender with a bit of sugar – it's going to make a lolly. Brrrrilliant.

SERVES **12**   CALS **80**   READY IN **190** MIN

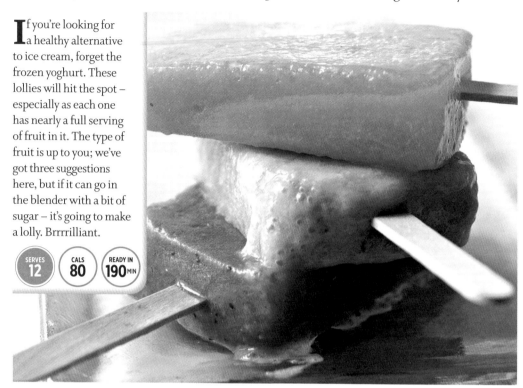

Mango-Chilli Blaster

INGREDIENTS
- 1 mango, chopped
- Juice of 1 lime
- 2 tbsp sugar
- Pinch cayenne pepper

METHOD Place the mango, lime juice, sugar and cayenne in a blender and purée, adding a bit of water if need be. Divide among 4 ice lolly holders and place in the freezer for 3 hours. To release the lollipops from the holders, run the bottoms briefly under warm water.

Boozy Banana Split

INGREDIENTS
- 2 ripe bananas, peeled
- 120ml low-fat milk
- 2 tbsp sugar
- 2 tbsp dark rum (optional)
- Pinch nutmeg

METHOD Place all the ingredients in a blender and puree, leaving the mixture slightly chunky if you like. A couple of spoons of rum will make this a barbecue star turn. Divide among 4 ice lolly holders and place in the freezer for at least 3 hours.

Strawberries and Cream

INGREDIENTS
- 400g strawberries
- 2 tbsp sugar
- 2 tbsp cream
- Juice of ½ lemon or lime

METHOD Blend all of the ingredients together until puréed. If you don't like seeds, strain them out through a fine sieve and discard. Divide the mixture between 4 ice lolly holders and leave in the freezer for at least 3 hours. Ideal for Wimbledon watching.

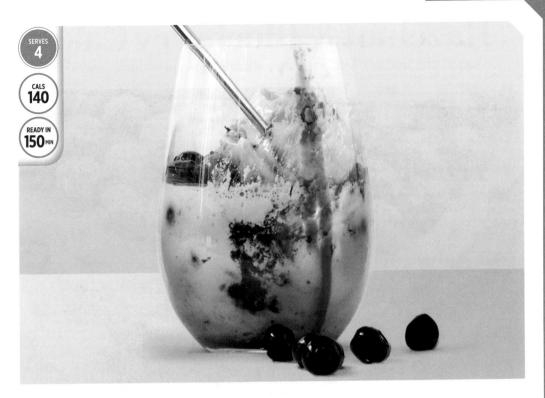

SERVES
4

CALS
140

READY IN
150 MIN

Skinny Panna Cotta

With just one simple savvy ingredient swap, this calcium-rich dessert is back on the menu

Panna cotta needn't cost you your figure – just follow our ingenious recipe and swap the cream for low-fat buttermilk. A single serving also provides 25 per cent of your RDA of calcium and the blueberries are rich in antioxidants. You just cotta try it.

INGREDIENTS
- 50g sugar
- 350g frozen blueberries, thawed
- 125ml condensed milk
- 360ml low-fat buttermilk
- 2 tsp lemon juice
- 1 tsp unflavoured gelatin
- Zest of 1 lemon

METHOD

1 Pour the evaporated milk into a small saucepan. Sprinkle in the gelatin and leave to sit for about 5 mins, while the gelatin softens. Next put the pan on a medium-low heat to cook, whisking constantly until the gelatin dissolves, then add the sugar. Stir it all in before removing from the heat.

2 While that cools, get another bowl and whisk the buttermilk and lemon zest and juice. Then add the milk mix, stirring constantly.

3 Now divide your blueberries between four glasses and pour over the mix. Finally, put them in the fridge for 2 hours to set before serving.

Hazelnut & Blueberry Cake

Go nuts for this healthy sweet. So pretty, you might not want to eat it... Just kidding!

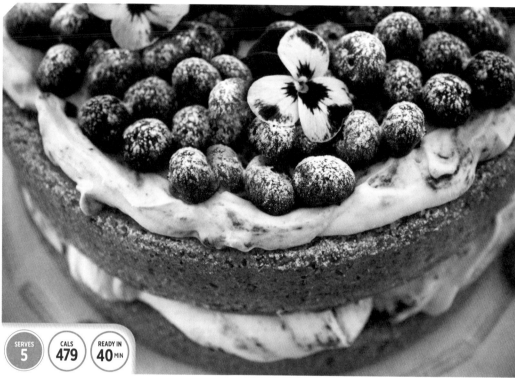

SERVES **5** CALS **479** READY IN **40** MIN

Spelt is your low-GI go-to when you fancy a spot of baking – it's lower in calories but higher in protein than regular flour. With protein-packed hazelnuts mixed in, we're talking about a tasty cake that doesn't result in a massive sugar spike after you've scoffed it. All of this goodness is topped with antioxdant-rich blueberries – making this cake this year's winner of the Great British Belly-Off.

INGREDIENTS
- 60g hazelnuts
- 130g soft unsalted butter
- 110g white spelt flour
- 1 teaspoon baking powder
- 2 large free-range eggs
- 65g honey (or golden caster sugar)
- 65g maple syrup
- Finely grated zest of ½ large unwaxed lemon
- 175g fat-free fromage frais
- 1 tablespoon honey
- ½ tablespoon sugar-free blueberry jam
- Handful of blueberries
- Violas to decorate (optional)

METHOD

1 Preheat oven to 180°C. Grease and flour two 20cm loose-bottomed sandwich tins. Toast hazelnuts for 5-7 mins. Leave to cool for 2 mins before rubbing off most of the skins. Whizz in a food processor.

2 Sift flour and baking powder into a large bowl and beat in all the other ingredients using an electric hand mixer. Bake for 25-30 mins until the cakes are golden and risen. Leave them to cool for 5 mins in the tins.

3 Lightly whip the fromage frais until thick, drizzle in honey and whisk again until incorporated, then marble the jam carefully through it. Trim the tops of the cakes so you have a flat surface to decorate. Spoon over most of the marbled honey filling, and put the second cake on top. Spread remaining filling on top of the second cake, then sprinkle on blueberries and violas.

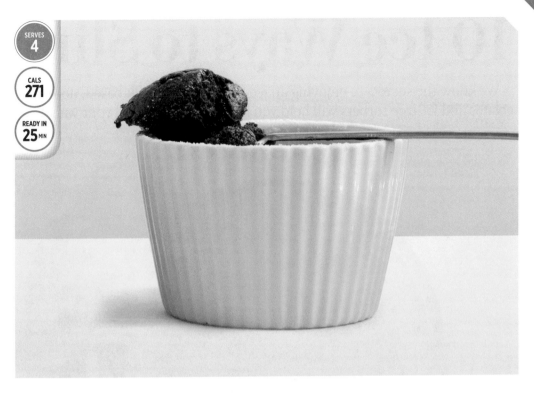

Lite Choc Mousse

An indulgent dessert without the guilt trip. Cook up a storm with this skinny chocolate treat

SERVES 4

CALS 271

READY IN 25 MIN

We've taken out the cream and popped in silken tofu (don't knock it till you've tried it, we promise it's not the same stuff you get in your Thai dinner!) for the same velvety texture with an added blast of calcium, vitamin E and hunger-busting protein. Chocolate heaven.

INGREDIENTS
- 340g soft silken tofu
- 125g fat-free Greek style yoghurt
- 170 melted dark chocolate chips
- 2 tsp vanilla extract
- 1 drop of almond extract
- 1 dark chocolate bar for garnish (optional)

METHOD

1 Blend or whisk the tofu, vanilla and almond extract together in a large bowl until smooth. Add the melted chocolate chips and blend again for 1 min. Scrape the sides with a rubber spatula and then blend again until your mixture is all combined.

2 Fold in the yoghurt until blended. Divide the mix among four ramekins, then pop them in the fridge until the mousse has set.

3 To garnish, draw a vegetable peeler along the edge of a bar of dark choc. Use the longer, narrower edge of your peeler to get skinny-minny shavings with (almost) zero calories.

10 Ice Ways to Slim

We know the secrets to enjoying an ice this summer: milk-based, no-egg gelatos and fat-free sorbets will help you keep your cool – and your waistline

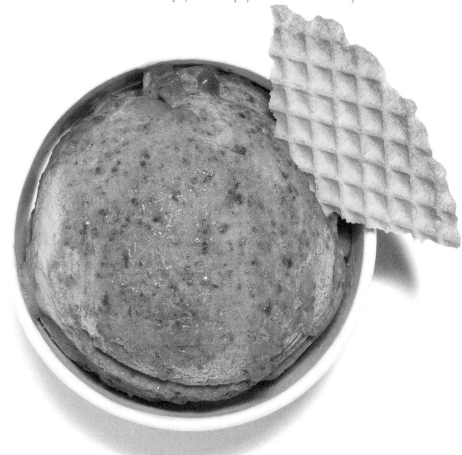

1: SLIM-DOWN STRAWBERRY SORBET
MAKES 12-15 SCOOPS | CALS 61 | PREP 20 MINS*

Sorbet syrup: 150g caster sugar • 50g runny honey • 3g leaf gelatine • Sorbet: 600g strawberries • Juice of 1 lemon to taste

Got your pinny on? For the syrup, bring 250ml water, the sugar and honey to the boil, then turn off the heat. Bloom the gelatine in cold water, drain, then stir into the hot sugar mix. Leave the syrup to cool. To make the sorbet, blend the berries with the syrup and lemon juice to taste. Freeze the mixture in an ice cream machine until ready to serve. Those tasty strawberries are high in fructose. If you eat this before a workout, the natural sugar will go directly to your muscles. Sweet, innit?

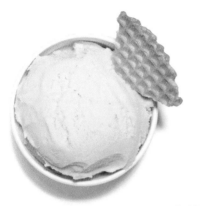

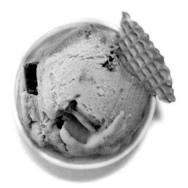

2: HUNGER-BUSTER PEANUT GELATO
MAKES 12-15 SCOOPS | CALS 156 | PREP 30 MINS

Base bianca (gelati base): 500ml whole milk • 140g whipping cream • 40g runny honey • 130g caster sugar 40g skimmed milk powder • 3g leaf gelatine • Gelato: 85g smooth peanut butter • 45g icing sugar

To make the base bianca gently heat the milk, cream and honey in a pan. In a bowl, mix the sugar and milk powder. When the pan steams, add the sugar mix as you stir. Simmer, and take off the heat. Soften the gelatine (the packet will tell you how), stir in and leave to cool. To make the gelato, blend in peanut butter and icing sugar and freeze in an ice-cream machine.

3: DR DIGESTION CHOC-MINT GELATO
MAKES 12-15 SCOOPS | CALS 145 | PREP 40 MINS

1 quantity base bianca, ice cold • 60g fresh mint, stalks and leaves included • 30g icing sugar • 40g dark chocolate (75% cocoa solids) • 20g coconut oil (optional, to thin the chocolate)

Make base bianca as before, but make ice cold. Blanch mint for 10 secs in boiling water, refresh for 20 more in iced water, then blend with dextrose and ¼ of base bianca until smooth. Sieve into the ice cream machine, then add the remaining base bianca. Churn until firm, melt chocolate with the coconut oil, cool and drizzle in. Firm in the freezer before serving.

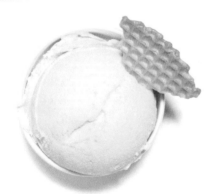

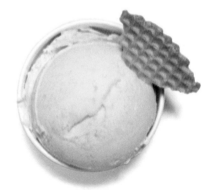

4: DE-BLOAT MELON SORBET
MAKES 12-15 SCOOPS | CALS 66 | PREP 20 MINS

1 quantity sorbet syrup • 1kg ripe orange-fleshed melon • Juice of 1 lemon to taste

Make syrup as before. Discard seeds from the melon and scoop out the flesh. Purée the fruit and pass it through a sieve to make a juice. Mix 650ml juice with syrup and lemon juice. Freeze until quite solid and dry-looking, then firm in the freezer for half an hour before serving.

5: SKINNY GRAPEFRUIT SORBET
MAKES 12-15 SCOOPS | CALS 64 | PREP 10 MINS

1 quantity sorbet syrup • 650ml freshly squeezed pink or red grapefruit juice (about 4-5 grapefruits)

Make the sorbet syrup, then mix with the juice of the grapefruit and pop into the ice cream machine until it becomes solid. Serve this fruity sorbet as a palette cleanser in between courses or pour a shot of vodka over it for a naughty – but not too naughty – treat.

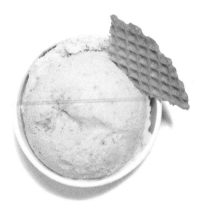

6: KICKSTART COFFEE GELATO
MAKES 12-15 SCOOPS | CALS 114 | PREP 25 MINS

1 quantity base bianca • 1 tbsp richly flavoured honey • 1 level tbsp ground coffee

Tell your metabolism to get cracking with caffeine. Make the base bianca as before, and leave to cool completely. Mix the ingredients and leave to stand for 30 mins, then churn. When the base is ready, add the honey and coffee and leave to stand for 30 mins before churning and freezing.

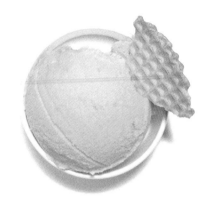

7: CLEANSING PEACH SORBET
MAKES 12-15 SCOOPS | CALS 72 | PREP 20 MINS

1 quantity sorbet syrup • 1kg ripe peaches with red-blushed skins • Juice of about 1 lemon to taste

Life's a peach with this big dose of vitamin C. Prepare the sorbet syrup as before. Blanch the peaches for 60 secs in boiling water. Cut the flesh off the stones, squeeze with lemon juice and puree. Press the puree through a sieve, and add to the syrup into your ice cream maker and freeze.

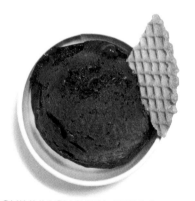

8: SKINNY CHOCOLATE SORBET
MAKES 12-15 SCOOPS | CALS 158 | PREP 20 MINS

50g cocoa powder • 200g caster sugar • 50g runny honey • 250g dark chocolate (70% cocoa solids) broken into pieces

A low-fat chocolate hit. Mix together cocoa and sugar. Stir in 500ml water bit by bit, then add honey. Bring to the boil, take off the heat when it bubbles, add chocolate and stir to mix. Cool to room temperature then blend with a hand-held blender. Freeze in an ice-cream machine.

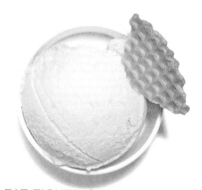

9: FAT-FIGHTING ALMOND SORBET
MAKES 12-15 SCOOPS | CALS 157 | PREP 40 MINS

1 quantity sorbet syrup • 200g blanched almonds • 60g caster sugar • 50g runny honey, • 1 tsp almond extract

Almonds are great for staving off cravings. Make syrup as usual. Blitz the almonds in a blender. Add 150ml water and grind for 5 mins more, add 850ml water. Let it sit for 20 mins, then sieve. Mix 650ml almond milk with sugar, sorbet syrup, honey and almond extract. Freeze.

10: FLAT-BELLY BERRY RICOTTA GELATO
MAKES 12-15 SCOOPS | CALS 118 | PREP 45 MINS

320ml whole milk • 50g honey • 130g caster sugar • 30g skimmed milk powder • 3g (bloomed) gelatine • 320g ricotta • 150g blueberries • 65g caster sugar • 1 tsp cornflour • 1 tsp almond extract

Bring the milk and honey to a boil. Mix 130g sugar with the milk powder and stir into the milk. Turn off the hob, add the (bloomed) gelatine and ricotta and blend. Cool to around room temperature then churn. Chop the berries, mix with 65g sugar and cornflour, bring to the boil, chill, then add the extract. Freeze until cold but not solid. Marble the berries through the ricotta and freeze for 30 mins. A study by Michigan University suggests blueberries help cut belly fat. Now that's super!

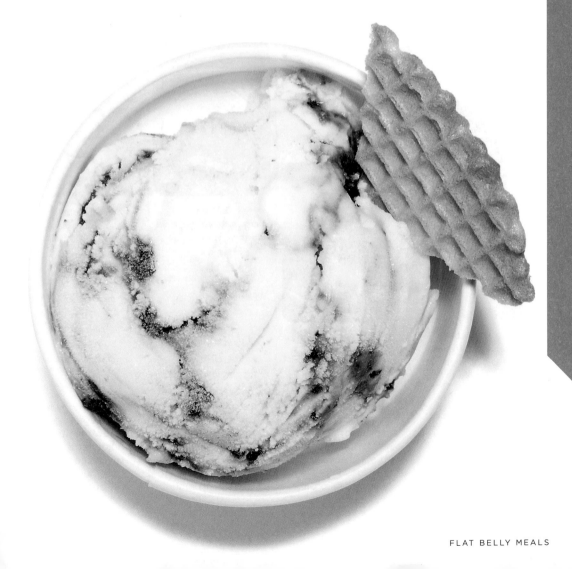

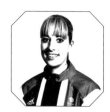

MY FLAT BELLY DIARY:

Charlotte Dujardin

Charlotte Dujardin OBE boasts a double gold in Olympic dressage
– what can we learn about how she fuels her winning streak?

MONDAY

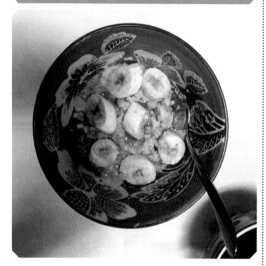

6:30am
*Porridge with banana
and semi-skimmed milk,
cup of tea*

8am
Lucozade Lite

1pm
*Salad with peppers
and tomatoes*

3pm
Cup of coffee, banana

7pm
Grilled salmon, asparagus

I leave the house early to get to the stables, so I don't always feel like eating first thing in the morning. But skipping breakfast isn't an option, as I need a lot of fuel for the day ahead. So I go for something quick but filling, like cereal, porridge or yoghurt.

TUESDAY

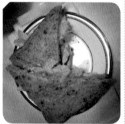

6:30am
*Mango, pineapple and grapes
with yoghurt, cup of tea*

8am
Coffee

1pm
*Wholemeal tuna sandwich,
cup of tea*

3pm
Cup of tea, banana

7pm
Homemade mushroom soup

I usually grab lunch on the go. Riding after a big meal gives me a stitch so if I'm going to be in the saddle in the afternoon I stick to something light. A sandwich or salad does the trick.

WEDNESDAY

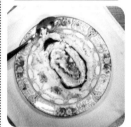

6:30am
*Special K with banana and
semi-skimmed milk*

8am
Cup of tea

1pm
Wholemeal chicken sandwich

7pm
Homemade parsnip soup

7:30pm
Meringue roulade

When I got my first dressage horse, I knew my fitness would play a role in my success. I'm conscious of what I eat but I do enjoy a post-dinner treat at least twice a week.

WORDS: AMELIA JEAN JONES. PHOTOGRAPHY: GETTY IMAGES.

THURSDAY

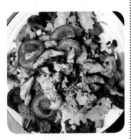

6:30am
Mango, pineapple and grapes with yoghurt, cup of tea

8am
Cup of tea

1pm
Chicken salad with spinach and tomatoes

3pm
Cup of coffee, banana

7pm
Homemade parsnip soup

I meet with my personal trainer to do two sessions a week. A mid-afternoon snack gives me the energy kick I need to for this.

FRIDAY

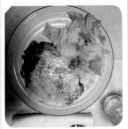

6:30am
Weetabix with banana and semi-skimmed milk, cup of tea

8am
Cup of tea, apple

1pm
Tuna salad with spring onions and tomatoes

3pm
Cup of coffee, banana

7pm
Lasagne and salad

I try to cook something healthy most evenings. It's great to come home after a boxercise class and treat myself to something stodgy.

SATURDAY

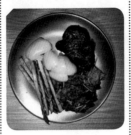

6:30am
Weetabix with berries and semi-skimmed milk, cup of tea

8am
Cup of tea

1pm
Chicken salad with peppers and tomatoes

7pm
Steak and vegetables

7:30pm
Glass of champagne

I don't often drink but if it's a special occasion, I'll go for a little champagne or schnapps with soda, and reduce some carbs to compensate.

SUNDAY

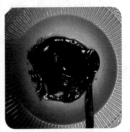

8am
Special K with banana and semi-skimmed milk

10am
Cup of coffee

1pm
Wholemeal tuna sandwich with salad

7pm
Homemade mushroom soup

7:30pm
Sticky toffee pudding

A day at the stables means up to six hours on a horse. I reward myself with the odd treat – you can't always be strict!

THE EXPERT VERDICT

Nutritional scientist Dr Christy Fergusson gives her take on our Olympian's food diary: "Charlotte's diet looks balanced overall. She eats plenty of fruit and vegetables, so that means she's getting more than the recommended five a day. But it does seem as if she might be more addicted to sugar than she's letting on. She should ditch the breakfast cereals for porridge in the morning and swap the bread in her sandwiches for quinoa, because these foods have a lower glycaemic load. She'll stay fuller for longer and won't feel the need to reach for the kettle to get a caffeine kick later on in the day.

"She seems to eat a lot of tropical fruit and should consider switching to berries to lower the sugar hit and to avoid dips in her energy levels.

"As for the puddings? Everyone has to have a treat. Try frozen bananas blitzed in a blender for a non-dairy, low-sugar sweet treat." Yum.

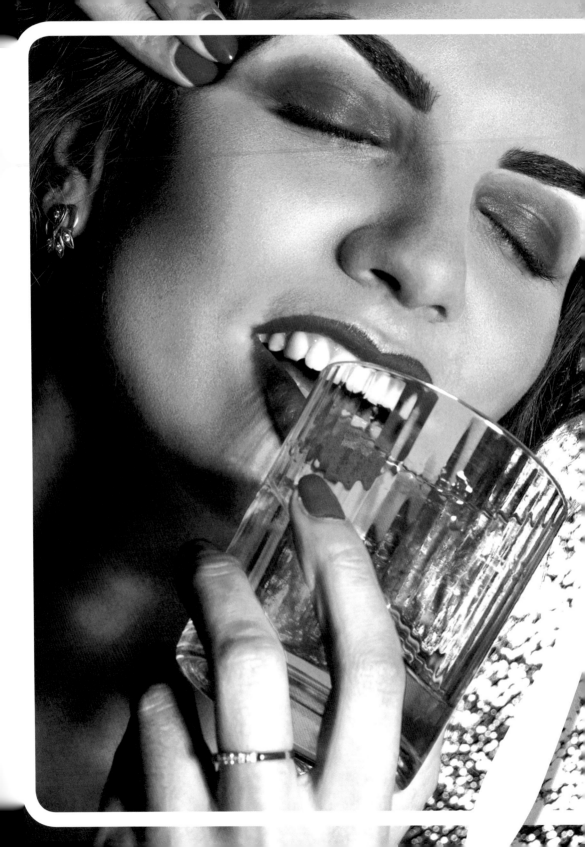

chapter 10

EAT OUT, LOSE WEIGHT

So all your hard work has paid off and you look pretty awesome in a party dress. Time to hit the town and celebrate – without undoing everything you've achieved. Sounds too good to be true? It isn't. We've got all the cheats to help you dodge the hidden fat hazards lurking in restaurant menus and make the best choices when it comes to your booze.

Outsmart any menu

Eating out can be a minefield when you're trying to lose weight, but with this guide to clever ordering, you can fend off a stealth attack on your eating plan

Not every menu choice is going to be as obviously lardy as Death by Chocolate. Which is a shame because dining out is one of the major threats to your weight loss goals. Research conducted at Cornell University in the US found the average diner underestimates how many calories they're eating by a whopping 38 per cent. Don't be one of them – we'll help you sort the nutritional wheat from the calorific chaff in these three eating-out scenarios...

1 THE LOCAL CAFE

1 PICK THE BEST OMELETTE
Go for feta and spinach for a nutritional gold star. Feta cheese has a third less fat than cheddar and spinach is packed with vitamins A and C. The eggs are a great source of protein and brain-boosting choline.

2 SAY BYE-BYE TO BAGELS
Watch out – a plain bagel packing 215 calories and over a gram of salt. Sneaky. Ask for a wholemeal muffin instead. On the upside, the salmon gives you a good dose of fat-burning omega-3 fats.

BREAKFAST

9.00-12.00 Hours

Served 9am-12pm

The Full Englis
Two fried eggs, t
pudding, baked

The Vegetarian
Two fried eggs, t
baked beans, mu

Omelette
Two-egg omelet
Cheddar cheese,

Eggs Benedict
Two poached eg

Bagel with smc
Toasted bagel wi

Organic porrid
With honey and

Pancakes
With maple syru

FROM THE B

Croissant
Banana bread
Fruit toast
Blueberry muf

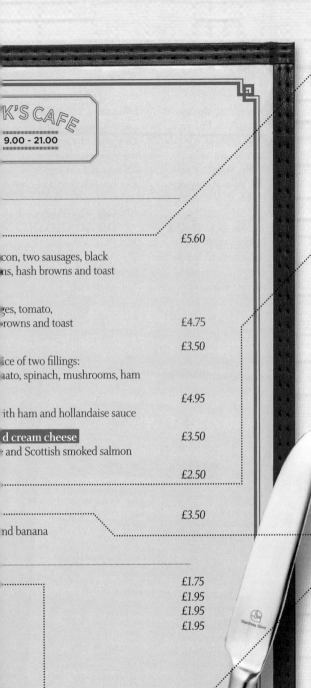

K'S CAFE
9.00 - 21.00

£5.60

...con, two sausages, black
...ns, hash browns and toast

...ges, tomato,
...rowns and toast £4.75

£3.50

...ice of two fillings:
...ato, spinach, mushrooms, ham

£4.95

...ith ham and hollandaise sauce

...d cream cheese £3.50
... and Scottish smoked salmon

£2.50

£3.50

...nd banana

£1.75
£1.95
£1.95
£1.95

3 STEER CLEAR OF THE SAUSAGE

A full English will pile on at least half your RDA of fat in one go. Instead, go for the veggie option. You'll get protein from the eggs and nutrients from the vegetables, minus the meat-eoric calorie count.

4 MAKE SURE YOU GET YOUR OATS

This is the best choice on the menu. Oats are low in fat and salt, plus they contain lots of soluble fibre, which helps lower your cholesterol levels. And, yes, the berry choice is the best one: you'll up your antioxidant, vitamin and fibre intake.

5 TURN PANCAKES DOWN FLAT

No surprises that these sweet, buttery treats don't make a healthy breakfast, but what you might not know is that a serving of maple syrup also contains 10% of your salt RDA – guaranteed to bring on the bloat.

6 CROSS OFF CROISSANTS

High in saturated fat, croissants are a big no-no. A slice of fruit toast is a filling, sweet alternative that brings only 0.9g of saturated fat. Get it with peanut butter for a dose of calcium, iron and 6g of protein to stay fuller for longer.

2 THE CURRY HOUSE

1 SLIM WITH THE SOUP
Dodge deep-fried appetisers and start with soup instead. Most are stock-based and packed with veg – so, more nutrients, fewer calories.

2 AVOID FALSE STARTERS
Pakoras are stuffed with veg or meat, then deep fried. At 200 calories a pop for the veggie version and around 300 if they have meat in, it's best to steer clear.

3 CURRY FAVOUR
Tandoori means cooked in a tandoor – a clay oven that heats up to 500°C, so no oil is necessary. If available, try tandoori fish – it's delicious and is under 500 calories.

4 TUCK INTO A TIKKA
It's lean chicken marinated in yoghurt and spices. But avoid tikka masala. Masala means "cream" in Hindi, which means "fat" in any language.

5 GET A GOOD DAAL
Find a way to make these stewed lentils a part of your meal – they're a low-fat source of protein and fibre. Plus, they'll keep you full to prevent snacking.

6 SAY NO TO NAAN
One naan has around 540 calories and 20g of fat, so consider sharing. Or opt for chapati minus the ghee (clarified butter) – it's roughly 110 calories and has 0.5g per slice.

7 GO VEGGIE OR GO HOME
Most Indian veg dishes are a better choice than heavy, meaty ones. The pulses add protein, and the veg increases nutrients. Watch out for creamy sauces, though.

THE RAJ

APPETISERS

Samosas £3.25
Vegetable or Meat

Onion Bhaji £3.50

Mulligatawny Soup £4.95
A mouthwatering recipe using the finest ingredients, flavoured with sharp tamarind and tangy tomatoes

Vegetable Pakoras £3.35
Spicy vegetables deep fried with garam flour

Chicken Pakoras £4.25
Diced chicken deep fried with spices and garam flour

HOUSE SPECIALS

Jaipuri £7.95
A potent fusion of peppers, onions, ginger, garlic, green chillies and a touch of coconut simmered in exotic jaipuri spices

Traditional Bhuna £7.50
A tasty condensed sauce with additional ginger and garlic

Chicken Tikka £9.95
Chicken marinated and cooked to perfection in the charcoal tandoori oven, served with rice

Rogan Josh £7.95
Lamb simmered until tender in a fusion of tomatoes, paprika and a host of spices

Murgh Makhani £7.95
Marinated chicken cooked in a creamy tomato and butter sauce with fragrant spices

Sambar Daal £7.95
A speciality from southern India, using the finest red lentils and flavoured with tamarind

THE RAJ

TANDOORI DISHES

Tandoori Chicken £9.95
Tandoori Lamb £10.95
Tandoori Fish £11.95
Tandoori Prawns £11.95

Sheesh Kebab £10.95
Fresh minced lamb mixed with chopped onion and fresh chillies

VEGETABLE DISHES

Karahi Vegetables £3.35
Mixed vegetables cooked traditionally with an abundance of fresh coriander and tomatoes

Chana Masala £3.75
Chickpeas cooked with tomatoes and chef's special sauce

Malaidar £3.95
Spinach puree simmered with lashings of green chilli and garlic, with a dash of fresh cream

Malabari Baingan £4.25
Aubergines cooked in a fragant coconut flavoured sauce with mustard seeds

SIDES

Naan bread £2.25
Garlic naan £2.95
Peshwari naan £2.95
Chapati £1.95
Tandoori roti £2.55
Paratha £2.95
Poppadom £1.15

Pilau rice £2.25
Mushroom rice £2.95
Special-fried rice £2.95
Spiced onions £2.95
Mango chutney £1.15
Raita £2.15
Seasonal salad £2.75

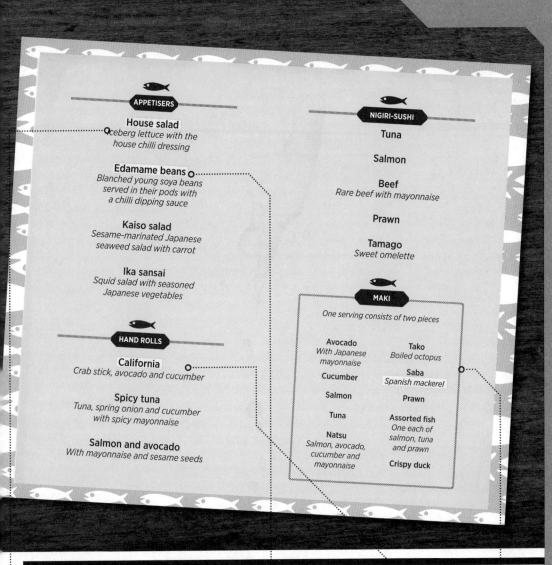

APPETISERS

House salad
Iceberg lettuce with the house chilli dressing

Edamame beans
Blanched young soya beans served in their pods with a chilli dipping sauce

Kaiso salad
Sesame-marinated Japanese seaweed salad with carrot

Ika sansai
Squid salad with seasoned Japanese vegetables

HAND ROLLS

California
Crab stick, avocado and cucumber

Spicy tuna
Tuna, spring onion and cucumber with spicy mayonnaise

Salmon and avocado
With mayonnaise and sesame seeds

NIGIRI-SUSHI

Tuna

Salmon

Beef
Rare beef with mayonnaise

Prawn

Tamago
Sweet omelette

MAKI
One serving consists of two pieces

Avocado
With Japanese mayonnaise

Cucumber

Salmon

Tuna

Natsu
Salmon, avocado, cucumber and mayonnaise

Tako
Boiled octopus

Saba
Spanish mackerel

Prawn

Assorted fish
One each of salmon, tuna and prawn

Crispy duck

3 THE SUSHI BAR

1 BREAK THE HOUSE

House salad sounds healthy but the lettuce offers very little nutritionally, plus 2 tbsp of oily dressing can pack up to 200 calories and 10g fat. Go for the seaweed salad, it's one of nature's most potent multivitamins.

2 MAKE MINE EDAMAME

High in protein and fibre and very low in calories, these beans make a good start to a meal. To avoid a sodium overload (which can lead to bloating), ask for your edamame without salt, then apply it yourself.

3 DREAM OF CALIFORNIA

Great news: the most popular menu item is also one of the most healthy. You'll get a dose of monosaturated fat from the avocado, and at just 300 calories per eight pieces, there's no need to feel guilty for filling your plate.

4 MAKE IT MACKEREL

Mackerel has twice the amount of heart-healthy, inflammation-reducing, cancer-fighting omega-3 fatty acids as salmon, making it one of the healthiest fish in the sea. We wish we'd found that out sooner, too.

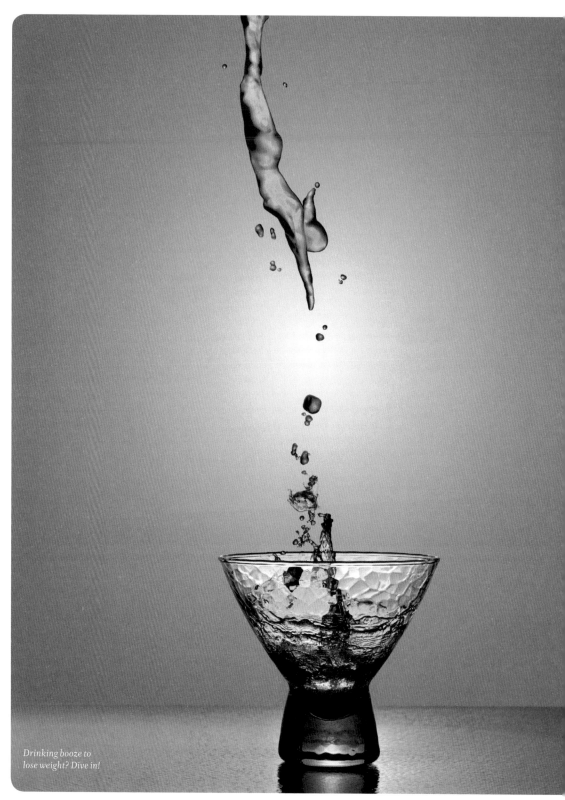

Drinking booze to lose weight? Dive in!

Boozing vs losing

You don't need to call last orders on drinking to lose weight. Drink smartly to make happy hour work for you with these alco-hacks

Good booze news just in: a study in the *Archives of Internal Medicine* found that moderate drinkers were less likely to gain weight than women who shunned the sauce completely. But before you crack open the Champagne to celebrate, remember: you need to drink smart. Here's what you need to know to make Friday night guilt free...

First up, what exactly is that Pinot Noir doing to your waistline? The average drink – beer, wine, snakebite and black (we're not judging) – is a combination of carbs, sugar and ethanol, aka pure alcohol. When it goes down, it makes a pit stop at your stomach, where some of the alcohol is absorbed into your bloodstream, (giving you buzz). Meanwhile, the carbs and sugar go the traditional digestive route, while ethanol, a toxin, is diverted to your liver.

Ethanol has no nutritional value, so your body burns it off first. So, any remaining calories in your stomach – whether they're from the margarita or the packet of cashew nuts you had with it – will probably be stored as fat – right around your middle. (Bear in mind that research published in *Physiology & Behavior* found that alcohol makes us focus on immediate pleasure and ignore the consequences, which often results in eating junk food). But until now, experts have struggled to nail down exactly why some women wind up with a beer belly, while others drink yet never seem to gain a pound.

The research in *Archives of Internal Medicine* found that women who had just one or two drinks a day were less likely to gain weight than non-drinkers. Even more surprisingly, they did it while consuming more calories overall (from food and drink) than heavy drinkers and teetotallers.

Here's how they managed to pull that off: researchers believe that the bodies of long-term, moderate drinkers adapt to metabolise alcohol differently. They burn more of the calories in the drink while digesting it, says Dr Lu Wang, the lead researcher. She found that, for women who drink up to two small glasses of wine a day, those calories simply don't end up as extra fat.

There is a catch. Save daily drinks for a big night out, and you don't qualify for the free calorie plan. "Your metabolism adjusts to the amount you normally drink," says Wang. So,

> Women who had just one or two drinks a day were less likely to gain weight than non-drinkers.

if you don't drink regularly, your body will store the extra calories from alcohol as fat.

For optimal fat-burning efficiency (not to mention health), it's good to give your liver a night off. Current government guidelines advise at least a couple of alcohol-free days per week – and not exceeding two to three units on the days you do drink.

It's advice worth sticking to. Evidence suggests moderate drinkers have healthier habits than teetotallers. "If you can moderate alcohol consumption you're more likely to behave in the same way with your eating habits," says Katie Peck, from the British Dietetic Association. "Teetotalers don't have the experience of having to control their drink levels, so they may be unable to adopt moderation when it comes to eating."

One more thing to bear in mind: the women in the study were served no more than two 125ml glasses of wine or two 35ml shots of spirits a day. In real life, you're more likely to be handed a glass big enough to accommodate a couple of goldfish – the average "small" serving of wine in British pubs is now 175ml. Order a large (250ml) and you're drinking a third of a bottle without being fully aware. (Keep that in mind at the next post-work drinks night).

And we're not much better when left to our own devices. "It's very easy to get the wrong measurement of alcohol," says Peck. "If you're at home, you don't have to adhere to the measurement guidelines that pubs and bars follow, so you might inadvertently pour too much." Yep, we've all been there.

The key to successful, safe moderate drinking is to slow down and pace yourself. Duck out of rounds if possible (especially if you're out with men – their bodies absorb

alcohol more slowly than us, damn them) and alternate each alcoholic drink with a glass of water. If you're having a big night out, prepare yourself by eating a good lunch – something with low-GI carbohydrates for

Order a large glass of wine and you're drinking a third of a bottle

energy, and protein to fill you up (a chicken or tuna salad sandwich is ideal).

Just before going out, eat a fibre-rich snack such as fruit, with yoghurt for protein. This will slow down alcohol absorption and keep you from ordering a mound of nachos before the barman has even brought your change.

Stick to these rules and, as the latest research proves, boozing doesn't have to be a fight against losing weight. You can actually do both at the same time (hello, multi-tasking) and be healthier too. We say cheers to that **WH**

BARMAN! MAKE MINE A...

Feel like an alcohol intellectual? Here's one more thing: we've put together these smart drink substitutions to help you save calories on a night out. Now that beats asking the barman for the nutritional info every time you order (awkward), or trawling the net the day before.

DRINK THIS | NOT THAT! | SAVE

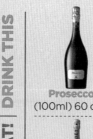
Prosecco
(100ml) 60 cals

Vodka & slimline tonic 58 cals

Mojito
215 cals

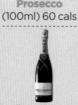
Moët & Chandon
(100ml) 83 cals

Jack Daniels & Coke 129 cals

Strawberry & mango margarita 350 cals

23 CALS

71 CALS

135 CALS

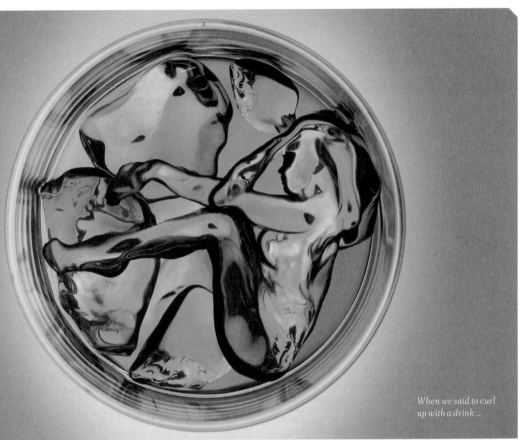

*When we said to curl
up with a drink...*

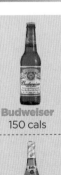	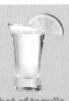				**TOTAL SAVE 550 CALS**
Budweiser 150 cals	**Shot of tequila** 115 cals	**Cosmopolitan cocktail** 170 cals	**Magners bottle** 205 cals	**Pimm's & Lemonade can** 167 cals	
Leffe Blonde 200 cals	**Shot of Drambuie** 165 cals	**Mai Tai cocktail** 310 cals	**Kopparberg bottle** 240 cals	**Gordon's Gin & Tonic can** 213 cals	
50 CALS	**50 CALS**	**140 CALS**	**35 CALS**	**46 CALS**	

RECIPES INDEX

INDEX

EDITOR-IN-CHIEF
Farrah Storr

EDITOR
Edie Mullen

ART DIRECTOR
Graeme Sapsed

SUB EDITORS
Rachelle Harry
Beth Wilson
Katherine Cowdrey

PRODUCTION
Roger Bilsland

TOTAL GYM INSPIRATION!

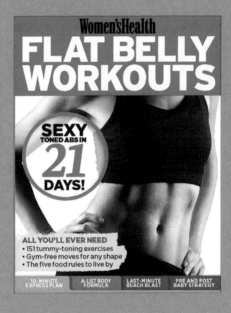

OVER
A YEAR'S
WORTH OF
WORKOUTS,
JUST £7.99!

Whether you've only got 10 minutes or a whole hour there's a plan here to guarantee you tighten your tummy and keep it that way. From perfecting your last-minute beach body to fitting workouts around pregnancy and motherhood, this book has all you need.

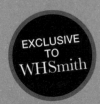

BETTER BODY SECRETS

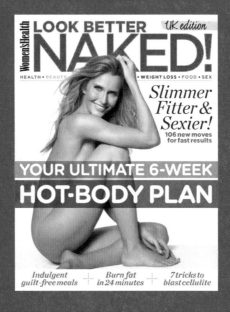

BETTER BARE BODY SECRETS FOR JUST £7.99!

Boost your body confidence overnight with the simple tips and tricks in this book. Get inspired by the *Women's Health* readers who have transformed their bodies, then follow their lead with a complete six-week exercise and nutrition plan, which combines simple workouts with delicious food to deliver fast results whatever your shape.

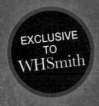